WAR

AGAINST

TIME

—ELEVEN ESSAYS

by
Sylvan Myron Elliot Shane

Foreword By

DR. STEVEN MULLER, President
The Johns Hopkins University

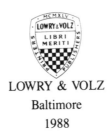

LOWRY & VOLZ
Baltimore
1988

Copyright, 1988
by
LOWRY & VOLZ, *Publishers*
1750 Union Avenue
Baltimore, Maryland 21211
U.S.A.

Library of Congress Cataloging in Publication Data
Library of Congress Catalog Card Number 88-80371
Shane, Sylvan Myron Elliot, 1918-   WAR AGAINST TIME—ELEVEN ESSAYS

1. Shane, Sylvan Myron Elliot, 1918-   2. Voyages and travels   I. Title.
DNLM: 1. Anesthesiology—Personal narratives. 2. Personal narratives.

ISBN 0-9601740-3-6

PRINTED IN THE UNITED STATES OF AMERICA

To My Children
Betty, Frank, Ruth, Nancy

"The written word alone flaunts destiny, revives the past, and gives the lie to death."

BOOKS BY THE AUTHOR

Out Of This World—Anesthetics And What They Do To You
Anesthesia For Frankie
The Practice of Balanced Anesthesia
Anesthesia—Thief of Pain
Handbook of Balanced Anesthesia
As I Saw It
A Method of Balanced Anesthesia in Surgery, Obstetrics and Dentistry
Principles of Sedation, Local and General Anesthesia in Dentistry
Routes Of A Dentist
Conscious Sedation For Ambulatory Surgery
From Pole To Pole and Between
War Against Time
Thou Shalt Not (A 3-act play)

CONTENTS

Chapter

FOREWORD

It is a special pleasure and privilege to offer this foreword to this latest work by Sylvan Shane. The same courage and spirit that emboldened him as a high school senior to gain entry into an operating room at The Johns Hopkins Medical Institutions to observe Dr. Walter Dandy; that led him to make the arduous trek across the Northwest Passage; and that inspired him to make the solo journey down the Baja Peninsula have prompted him to share with us a collection of eleven thoughtful essays which describe some of the most significant moments in his life.

With an appealing blend of candor and eloquence, Dr. Shane takes us with him into the Cameroons, across the Northwest Passage, and down the Baja. He provides us with keen insights into the intractable conflict between Arabs and Israelis as well as with the fine points of building a glass house. Understandably, the essay on "The Anesthesia Years at Johns Hopkins" is of special interest to me. Johns Hopkins has been fortunate to have the benefit of Dr. Shane's experience and expertise. His pioneering work on conscious sedation has had a significant influence on future generations of dentists and physicians.

Dr. Shane's work is touched throughout with humor and warmth, and his essays are a pleasure to read. At a time when many others of his age may be taking their retirement literally, Dr. Shane is facing new challenges and setting new goals. He is indeed a winner in the war against time.

Steven Muller
President
The Johns Hopkins University

PROLOGUE

On an Autumn afternoon I sat in Baltimore's Druid Hill Park and wrote of the meaning of retirement.

It is an inconspicuous, bright, cicada-chirping, September afternoon. The sunlight casts its slanting rays which reflect like dull mirrors off the fluttering leaves. It is warm enough to encourage the cicadas autumn symphony, but September has diminished the cadence. The rhythm is slower, the tone softer and more mellow and consonant with the yellow and crimson of the dogwood's hue.

The leaves sprout their grey hairs among the green and the grass harbors the graves of the fallen leaves. The leaves, like humans, are born in the Spring, strut through their heydays of Summer, and in the September of their lives turn from the green of middle age to the gold of Autumn's chill, then fall to their graves.

I sit in Druid Hill Park and become one with the leaves that, like myself, are retiring. I too, recall the heydays of my productive years. September was the start of kindergarten, high school, college and profession. There was never time to listen to the cicada's Autumn swan song. But I hear it now, and at last I sense my destiny, my finiteness, and I become one with the greying leaves. Many of my associate leaves who fluttered with me through the Summer have already fallen and lie in the grass. But clinging to my tree I continue to flutter in this multicolored Autumn, sensing at the same time the distant chill of Winter's long sleep.

One has to personally experience each season to fully appreciate its departure. I look back at the hours of study, the preparation of assignment papers, the "at last" sigh of graduation, the excitement of marriage, the mystery of a first born, the blunders and achievements of a profession, the thrill of exploring the world, and all those seasons suddenly coalesce into a single thought, as if in a dream, and I find myself retired in my park on an inconspicuous afternoon. I hear amidst the song of the cicadas the last period dismissal bell in high school since it's now 2:30. But now there's no homework, no struggle for a livelihood, no need to achieve that phantom called success. It's all behind me now.

I may not have heard the sounds of Spring nor the music of Summer, but the melodious symphony of the Autumn of my years accompanies the voice of the cicadas.

I sit in deep repose, thankful to be able to appreciate at last, the music that surrounds me, and to look with pleasantness to Winter's final ballad.

Sylvan M. Shane
2220 Old Taneytown Road
Westminster, Maryland

CHAPTER I

ATTEMPTING THE
NORTHWEST PASSAGE

Retirement is the time in one's life to explore remote areas of the planet. The Northwest Passage is an impossible ice choked route between the Atlantic Ocean and the Pacific, across Canada's High Arctic, far above the Arctic Circle where trees and grass are unknown; where the Eskimo and polar bear vie for their chief source of food, the seal; where a thousand ships tried and failed to negotiate the ice; where hundreds of intrepid explorers froze to death in the ice trap not far from the North Pole.

This is where I decided to requite one of my dreams.

On August 29, 1986, I left Baltimore by air, flew to Edmonton, Canada, then by charter flew North in a propeller-driven plane to a frozen, isolated outpost known as *Resolute*. This was a weather station in a remote frozen region of the Arctic high above the Arctic Circle.

The flight from Edmonton, Canada, to Resolute required 4 hours. Resolute is a Harbor village on the southern end of an island known as Cornwallis Island located on the Barrow Strait which is on the 75th parallel, about 200 miles south of the North Magnetic Pole. The typical northern sky became even more "northern" as the plane flew ever northward. Soon snow made its appearance 20,000 feet below, after which all the trees said their farewell and the land below became a lonely, desolate wasteland, barren of trees and grass; only stony earth, snow-covered hills, and patches of floating ice in the many rivulets, lakes and streams far below.

After 4 hours on this Northwest Territorial Airways propeller plane, the sky clouded up and the stewardess announced we were preparing to land. The stewardess had never been this far north before since this was a chartered flight, specifically for this Northwest Passage expedition. I wondered if the pilot had ever been here before. Soon the plane descended out of the clouds, and snow and ice-covered land appeared once again. No sign of life. Only barrenness everywhere and in all directions. As the plane descended closer to the ground the first sign of civilization was a series of one-story, tin shacks with navigation towers blinking red lights. The plane touched ground on an island so remote it was difficult to locate it on the map.

All my Arctic wool and parkas were in my baggage in the plane's hold. I was wearing the summer suit I wore when I departed the heat of Baltimore's August. The airport was a makeshift tin shack of a building with the word "RESOLUTE" on the sign above the entrance. When the plane door opened the temperature was below zero, the wind was howling and the snow bit into my face. Between descending the plane's stairway and running a 100-yard dash across the airfield to the tin shack I almost froze. The inside of the tin building reminded me of the tin building along the Trans-Siberian Railway when I had to dash from that train for food in the midst of winter in Siberia.

I then had to leave the warmth of this reception building and make another dash to a waiting bus that was at least vintage 1950 which was to escort the passengers to the waiting ice-breaker vessel, located on the other side of Cornwallis Island.

Soon, in the distance I could see the vessel, the World Discoverer, which was anchored about a mile offshore since there was no pier or dock.

Fortunately, the launch which held 40 people, was semi-closed for the wild ride on the wind-swept Arctic waters. I sat between two fat ladies who helped keep me warm during this 15-minute ride to the vessel which was to be my home for the next month.

I keep mentioning the sky here in the Arctic. I think the best description is that the sky is moody and brooding in its wind-swept grandeur. Daylight persists almost to midnight in this land of the midnight sun. In summer the sun never sets. It reaches the horizon, paints the sky in a symphony of exquisitely blended colors, rides the horizon through the night, and when it reaches the eastern part of the heavens, it proceeds to rise again, heralding the start of a new day. One can, therefore, enjoy an all-night sunset. Very few in this world ever have the privilege of experiencing this unique aspect of God's creation. To experience and appreciate such sublime artistry there must have been implanted in mankind the ability to interpret all this as art in its highest form.

During the first night of this voyage the ship sailed eastward through Barrow Strait, then turned south and entered the Admiralty Inlet. We were sailing in a part of the world that is far north of the Arctic Circle, about 500 miles north, far above the so-called tree line, where no trees or vegetation ever grows, and where there are a multitude of small and large

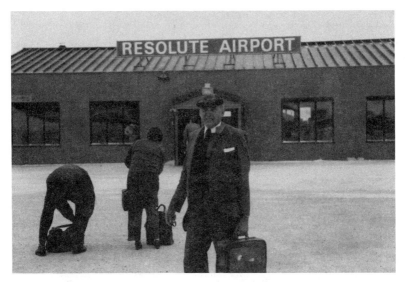

Arriving at Resolute near the North Magnetic Pole. Resolute Airport was an ice-bound, electrically-heated, tin structure.

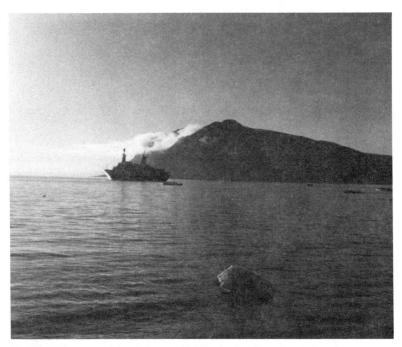

The World Discoverer waits offshore amidst floating ice, for arriving passengers.

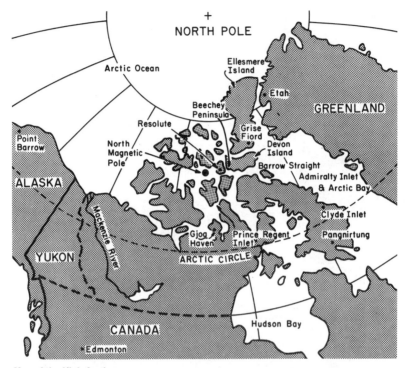

Map of the High Arctic.

bone-bare, snow-and-ice-covered islands through which the ship maneuvers to find scattered Eskimo outposts.

The ship's captain sounded an alert. A polar bear was sighted on one of the large ice floes. Everyone dashed for his camera and parka and headed for the port side of the ship. Outside on the decks it was biting cold, and there he was, a 1400-pound polar bear in his natural habitat, not swimming in Baltimore's make-shift Arctic zoo.

The United States and Canada have signed an agreement to limit the number of polar bears that can be hunted and killed in a given year. A polar bear skin is worth about $5,000. The hair on the skin of a polar bear consists of hollow tubes, like minute drinking straws. The air tubes form the highly efficient insulation barrier not only for the bear but for the Eskimo, since he uses polar bear skins for his pants and boots.

The ship maneuvered slowly towards the ice floe and kept circling it so everyone on board could get a good Kodachrome shot of the bear.

The word Eskimo means "eater of raw meat". He does not like that word and prefers being called "INUIT" which means "peoples." INUK is one person or one Eskimo. The Northwest Passage is the shortest route between Europe, the Atlantic, the Pacific, and Japan. The Canadian Government is now conducting studies on the effect of freighters and oil tankers on the wildlife in this passage such as whales, polar bears, foxes, seals, and other animals. Since the discovery of the Northwest Passage by Raul Amundsen in 1906, over 500 ships have attempted to navigate this passage but only 36 have been successful. The others had to turn back because of the unpredictability of the ice, whether in summer or winter.

On the afternoon of September 1st we dropped anchor one mile off shore at a God-forsaken, remote, outpost in the midst of floating ice, surrounded by snow-clad hills. On the distant shore were low one-story shacks and bungalows, and through binoculars could be seen scattered garbage, an unpaved road and oil-storage tanks. The place was called Arctic Bay. It was located at the end of a pocket, a branch off the Admiralty Inlet at the northern extremity of Baffin Island, high in the Arctic where night reigns without a speck of sunlight for three months of the year. At this time daylight had its turn.

Into zodiaks we climbed, wrapped snugly in layers of sweaters, covered by a down-stuffed water-proof red parka with the insignia NORTHWEST PASSAGE sewn on to the left arm. My head was covered in two layers of itchy wool, plus the red parka hood, and my hands were cloaked in silk gloves covered by fur-lined leather gloves. Four pairs of wool socks covered my feet which fit too tightly in my high rubber boots. A life jacket topped all of this insulation, and around my neck were two cameras.

The zodiak with ten passengers sped through the frigid Arctic waters to the rock-strewn shore, covered with seal carcasses, stones, and general debris. The shore was crowded with wide-eyed Eskimo children of all ages, some of whom had never seen a modern ocean-going vessel. We were like strangers from another planet descending en masse to their shore. The entire Eskimo settlement lined the shore to observe our dramatic arrival from the monster vessel anchored far out in the bay, the first passenger vessel they had ever seen.

This small community of Eskimos on the rocky shore of nowhere surprised me at every turn. Firstly, there is an ultra-modern school, built a year ago, with funds provided in part by the Bromfman family of Canada, the whiskey distillers, who have provided funds for so many projects in Israel. There was also a new gymnasium. The school is built on stilts and rests two feet above ground since the entire area sits on permafrost. If the

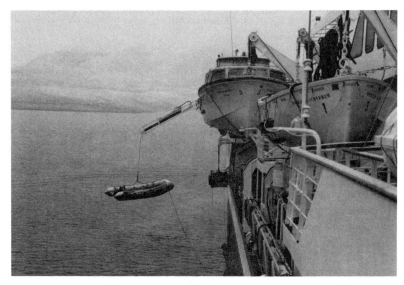

Upper) Zodiak being lowered into Ocean Lower) Passengers boarding the Zodiak

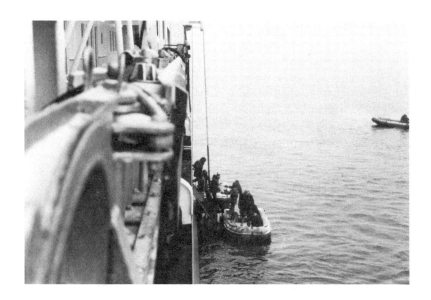

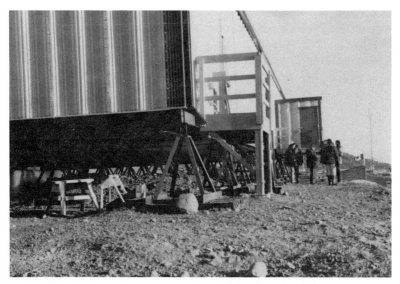

Eskimo homes must rest on stilts above ground, otherwise the heat from the floor of the home would melt the permafrost foundation causing the home to topple.

school sat on a concrete foundation, the heat from the building would melt the permafrost, the pipes would fracture and the building would topple over. All the bungalow-type houses and single-story shacks are on stilts to prevent melting of the permafrost, since the climate is freezing even in summer.

A head of lettuce costs $6.95 in United States dollars. This gives some idea of the cost of living in the Arctic. Where do the Eskimos get this kind of money? Most are on welfare, and like American Indians on the reservations in Arizona and New Mexico, the Canadian government foots the bill. Few of the anti-killing or anti-hunting laws that pertain to white men affect the Eskimo. They are like a protected species. But the price the Eskimo pays for this protection and white-man support is poison to Eskimo culture. Eskimo culture is one of hunting and gathering. Now he is subject to the laws of Canadian "civilization" and that means Coke, Wheaties, Pepsi, Snickers, TastyCake, U.S. and Canadian TV (one TV Station is received by satellite). The children suffer tooth decay and other ills brought on by an excess of white flour and sugar in the diet. There is wide unemployment. The government provides a nurse practitioner who acts similarly to the barefoot doctor in China. A dental technician, a female, is the community's dentist. She fills teeth, cleans and extracts them and even places stainless steel crowns. If someone is seriously ill, in the opinion of the nurse, she radios for a medivac plane which must fly in from headquarters in Frobisher Bay located 1,000 miles away at the southern tip of Baffin Island which is still 300 miles north of Labrador, far above Hudson Bay. And if the weather is anti-airplane, which it mostly is, too bad for the ill patient.

Much of the employment, and the reason for the airstrip, and boat dock, both of which are located 20 miles farther up on the island, is the presence of a lead and zinc mine, which I visited, known as Nanisivik. This is a unique, underground mine. The Canadian Government decided to invest in building this semi-modern outpost since Eskimos were a permanent source of labor. To depend on white men to live permanently in this supremely beautiful, but perpetual deep freeze was undependable.

The mine is the only one of its kind in the world where the temperature is constantly five degrees below zero Farenheit. Normally temperatures in deep underground mines is constant at 58 degrees, like a cellar. But this mine is dug under the centuries-old permafrost which is old, old compacted ice, and the ice surrounding the mine and mine shafts maintains this freezing temperature. This place was made to order for an Eskimo.

In summer the temperature at the entrance to the mine might be the same as the outside temperature which might rise to 33 degrees, just above freezing. To prevent the permafrost from melting and causing a collapse of the mine entrance, they have to close off the entrance to keep the coldness in, like closing windows in summer to keep the cold, air conditioning indoors.

Lead, zinc, and silver are found in abundance in the ore. Normally mining drills use water on drill tips to keep them cool. But no water can be used since it would freeze. So they drill dry and this creates excessive dust which contains lead, a lethal contaminant. They developed an immense vacuum system on the drills to suck in the dust. The ore is crushed in giant stone crushers and fed by a mile-long, rubber conveyer belt to freighters. The freighters carry the ore through the eastern entrance to the Northwest Passage. The freighters then sail through Lancaster Sound in Baffin Bay, through Davis Strait around the southern tip of Greenland and into the Atlantic Ocean and on to Belgium where the crushed ore is smelted into zinc, lead and silver.

Freighters can get into this area only two months of the year, August and September, because of the ice. The mine keeps producing during the ice-bound months and the crushed ore is stored in 100-pound bags in a storage area larger than two football fields.

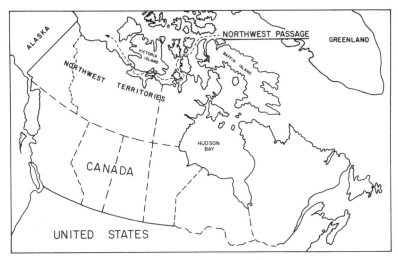

The dotted line shows our proposed route through the Northwest Passage.

The unhappy aspect of this mine which has been producing ore for about 20 years is that the ore will be all dug out by 1991, five years hence, and the place will become a ghost town. The white bosses, accountants, secretaries, and foreman will all go south to Canadian cities and the unemployed Eskimo will remain in the frigid temperatures that he loves so much.

On the third day out we arrived at Beechey Island, a tiny nameless place on the map of Canada's Northwest Territories. It is attached by a thin peninsula to Devon Island, a major island north of Baffin Island, lying in Lancaster Sound, the route of the Northwest Passage.

Why did the ship drop anchor here? The place is historic and the following is the sequence of events which warranted this special visit.

The search for the Northwest Passage has been a tempting carrot for more than a century. Before the discovery of oil, the need for spices, diamonds, and silks from the Orient was the beckoning carrot. Today it's oil and minerals such as zinc, lead, mercury, silver and gold and now uranium. If a ship leaving Europe cannot negotiate this Northwest Passage it originally had to go the length of North and South America, around treacherous Cape Horn and then across the fat belly of the Pacific at the Equator. Today the trip is somewhat shortened by the Panama Canal. But the Northwest Passage was shorter by months in the 1800's and today with the Panama Canal cutting out South America, it is shorter by a few weeks, but it is still too long a route to the Orient. The Northwest Passage would save 8,700 miles.

In 1845 the maritime nations like Britain directed their sailors to somehow find that Northwest Passage, and all sorts of expeditions set out. Most of them were either lost or frozen in the ice. To this day only 36 ships have ever gotten through the Northwest Passage to the Pacific. The ship I'm on will be the 37th in all history if we can break through the ice barriers which we run into every day. The Canadian Coast Guard has been so kind and generous with us. They have a real ice breaker which has been following us in the event our ship can't break through the ice or in the event we become iced in. Our ship is constructed for going through ice but it is not a true ice breaker.

In the year 1000 the Vikings got one-quarter way through, and remains of their ships tell the fatal story in the ice. In 1497 John Cabot sailed from Bristol, England, but failed off the Newfoundland Coast.

In 1527 a British captain named Thorue failed. In 1576 Martin Frobisher tried and failed. They named a bay for him.

In 1585 John Davis tried and they named Davis Strait for him.

In 1610 Henry Hudson got as far as Hudson's Bay. He failed.

In 1616 William Baffin got as far as we anchored today. He, too, failed. A Bay was named after him.

In 1700's too many men were lost in the previous century so no one attempted it.

In 1818 John Ross failed and had the Ross Strait named after him.

In 1819 W. E. Parry got as far as Melville Peninsula and they named Parry Bay after his failure. He carried a piano on his ship and when frozen in the ice he carted his piano onto land, and his cart wheel tracks are in the ice today. Parry was the explorer who, upon arriving at the small island attached by a peninsula to the larger Devon Island, sent one of his men ashore to investigate it. Parry named it Beechey Island after a British artist named Beechey, in the hope that the artist would paint Parry's portrait without charge. The largest channel from Baffin Bay in the East to the Beaufort Sea in the West is the Parry Channel.

In 1829 John Ross tried again, but failed.

In 1845 Sir John Franklin, and 128 of his crew were frozen in the ice close to where I went ashore on Beechey Island. The gravestones of some of his men stand alone in the ice, the inscriptions on the stone are almost completely eroded. One inscription read:

> "Sacred to the memory of John Torrington who departed this life
> Jan. 20, 1846 aboard HMS Terror. Age 20 years."

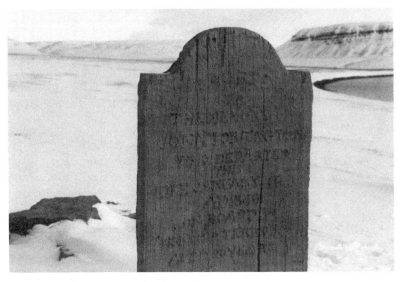

Upper) The Beechey Island gravemarker of John Tarrington who froze to death attempting the Northwest Passage in 1845.

Lower) The graves of some of the 128 men of Sir John Franklin's 1846 expedition who froze to death at this site on Beechey Island. Our ship and an ice breaker ride anchor in the distance.

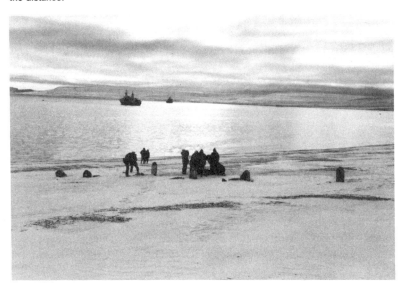

I was able to photograph the graves as I stood all bundled up in multiple sweaters, parka, head all covered, and warm in rubber boots, and my stomach full of peaches, guava fruit, sliced pineapple, soft-boiled egg whites, and sardines.

I stood facing these graves on the ice-covered shore of this small Beechey Island, surrounded by the sea on one side with its floating small icebergs, and on the other by barren, sullen, silent ice-covered hills. Those interred in the icy earth stood here as I stood and saw the same sight of unspeakable beauty. There is a mood that the Arctic conveys. A mood of utter silence, untouched by civilization. And somehow you sense the meaning of eternity in this vast, white, cold land of silence that refuses to let man penetrate beyond a certain point. How comforting that Canadian ice breaker looked riding anchor next to our ship.

For a moment, as I stood next to their graves, I felt the utter and complete isolation and the Arctic chill that they felt. I pictured their vessel, a wooden ship with only canvas sails for power. Motors were not invented in 1845, the year anesthesia was discovered. I stood there alone, far away from other passengers who were ferried by rubber zodiak boats from our ship anchored a mile away in the bay. I could appreciate the pristine beauty of this treeless Arctic wilderness that knows no flowers or trees; that simply sits here untouched since creation in its white, undulating icy splendor. The exquisite beauty of this place, if an artist or a Kodachrome could reproduce it, would be almost unbelievable. I stood there, alone, and gazed and gazed until tears blurred my vision. I appreciated with thankfulness the unique privilege I was experiencing in being able to be at this seldomly seen work of the Creator's artistic brush. Words are inadequate to describe the inner feelings which well up within a person. I had earphones under my parka hood and listened to music that I had previously recorded so that this experience would not only be captured in film, but with music as well.

Cold creeping into my boots forced me to go back to the zodiac which whisked me back to "mother" ship where it was warm and comfortable. From the ship's window I could continue to gaze at the blue sky, sea, and ice-covered mountains.

Sir John Franklin and his 128 sailors were all frozen to death right in this part of the beginning of the Northwest Passage and they named not a bay but the entire area for him, now known as the District Of Franklin which includes Victoria Island, Prince Of Wales Island, Somerset and Baffin Island, a distance of 2,000 miles, east to west, comprising almost the entire Northwest Passage.

Signs of TB, possible lead poisoning found in bodies from 1845 Arctic trek

9/24/86

> **Most of the experts said it couldn't be done.**
>
> **LARRY ANDERSON**
> **Radiologist**

EDMONTON, Alberta (AP) — The bodies of two English seamen who died 140 years ago in a doomed expedition to the Arctic were exhumed this summer and autopsies show signs of tuberculosis and possible lead poisoning, scientists said yesterday.

The bodies of a seaman, John Hartnell, 25, and a Royal Marine, William Braine, 33, had partly decomposed in their icy tomb but still were identifiable, a team of Canadian and U.S. scientists said at a news conference in Edmonton.

Sir John Franklin, a veteran Arctic explorer, and 128 handpicked officers and men perished mysteriously in 1845 on their expedition to find a northwest passage through what is now the Canadian Arctic.

Their disappearance prompted one of history's largest rescue searches from 1848 to 1859, which resulted in discovery of a northwest passage and the location of a graveyard and relics of the Franklin expedition in Canada's northern wastes.

Franklin's two well-equipped ships, the Erebus and the Terror, never were found.

Scientists continue to try to piece together the reasons for Franklin's failure. Owen Beattie, an anthropologist at the University of Alberta, first led a team to the Beechey Island graveyard in 1984. The island lies 745 miles from the North Pole near Lancaster Sound and was Franklin's first winter camp.

Mr. Beattie's first expedition uncovered the perfectly preserved remains of Petty Officer John Torrington, a 20-year-old boiler stoker aboard one of Franklin's two ships. His body, buried in an ice-filled coffin, was exhumed and an autopsy indicated he probably died of pneumonia.

Mr. Beattie returned this summer with a second team, including two radiologists, Larry Anderson of Park Nicollet Medical Center in Minneapolis, Minn., and Dr. Derek Notman. The Americans said they believed they were the first to use X-ray equipment in the high Arctic. They had gained experience by X-raying mummified bodies entombed in the Egyptian pyramids.

"Most of the experts said it couldn't be done," Mr. Anderson said. "The working conditions were not what we're used to back home."

The scientists said bad weather probably forced fellow crewmen to keep the bodies of Hartnell and Braine on board the Erebus for as long as a week before burial.

"The bodies were decomposed somewhat but they were recognizable," said the team pathologist, Roger Amy.

The two crewmen were buried without shoes or pants, unlike the fully clothed Torrington, probably because of their difference in rank, Mr. Amy said.

"Autopsies indicated signs of tuberculosis and possible lead poisoning from the canned food Franklin carried. There was no evidence of scurvy, a disease common to sailors and caused by a lack of vitamin C.

The men were very thin but it was unclear whether they starved to death, Mr. Beattie said.

The investigation will continue in the laboratory as team members pore over samples of hair and fingernails brought back from Beechey.

"We are still not sure what caused this disaster," said Mr. Beattie. He said it would take at least a year to publish findings in academic journals.

Recent 1986 BALTIMORE SUN report of Franklin's Northwest Passage expedition of 1845 in which 128 men perished. This report details the exhuming of John Tarrington's perfectly preserved body. The scientists discovered signs of tuberculosis and lead poisoning.

Following the disappearance of his ships, many search parties were sent out by the British Government to find these men.

It wasn't until 1947 that 69 skeletons were found and identified as men on the fatal Franklin expedition.

So far no one had successfully gotten through this invincible passage.

In 1871 Charles Hall failed.
In 1880 Great Britain turned the entire area over to Canada.
In 1881 Greeley failed.
In 1898 Otto Sverdrup, a Swede, failed.

But in the year 1903 a great Norwegian Arctic explorer named Roald Amundsen set out to find the Northwest Passage. He found it. It took three years since he had to winter-over at a point in the passage known as Gjoa Haven. By 1906 he was the first man in history to have successfully sailed this passage. Amundsen was also the first man in history to have reached the South Pole on December 14, 1911, beating the explorer Robert Falcon Scott to the Pole by a month.

Sir John Franklin and his men left messages behind in lonely stone cairns. The messages were left when they had lost hope and knew that death was waiting. One of the messages written by James Fitzjames, captain of H.M.S. Erebus after Franklin's death aboard the ship, read as follows:

> "April 25th, 1848—H.M. ships Terror and Erebus were deserted on 22 April, 5 leagues NNW of this (cairn) having been beset (in the ice) since 12th Sept. 1846, the officers and crew consisting of 105 souls under the Command of Captain F.R.M. Crozier landed here in Lat. 69° 37′ 42″ N. and Longitude 98° 41′W . . . Sir John Franklin died on the 11th June 1847, and the total loss by death in the Expedition has been to this date 9 officers and 15 men."
>
> James Fitzjames, Captain
> H.M.S. Erebus

This document contains all that will ever be known about the 128 men who sailed with Franklin to seek the Northwest Passage.

> William Smith in his book *Northwest Passage* wrote: ". . . the courageous men who challenged the Arctic . . . accepted defeat unflinchingly, but they wanted someone, anyone, to know what they had done and why they had died. The Arctic has often pushed men to their physical and mental limits; stripped them of all civilization, and driven them to an animal-like existence in which the frenzied hunt for food and warmth were the only realities. But the starved and diseased shadows that stalked the north also carried a spark, a nobility, that does honor to us all."

Roald Amundsen in 1901 at age 28 brought a herring boat named Gjoa. He installed a 13-horsepower kerosene engine, and with six other men set sail for the Northwest Passage on June 16, 1903. He followed the west coast of Greenland as Baffin had, entered Lancaster Sound like Parry and followed Sir John Franklin's course down Peel Sound. At Gjoa Haven on King William Island he spent 19 months making scientific observations around the magnetic North Pole, waiting for the ice to open. The ice thawed sufficiently and on August 13, 1905, his tiny ship sailed through Simpson Strait, Dease Strait, Coronation Gulf, Dolphin and Union Strait, then through a gulf which now bears his name, Amundsen Gulf, and on August 26, 1905 he sighted Nelson's Head on the southern tip of Banks Island, the entrance to the Beaufort Sea.

Amundsen wrote: "It seemed as if the Gjoa understood that the hardest part of the struggle was over, she seemed so wonderfully light in her movements."

The Northwest Passage had finally been conquered, although the Gjoa had to spend another winter in the ice of the Beaufort Sea at the mouth of the MacKenzie River off the north coast of Alaska.

Roald Amundsen emerged into the Pacific Ocean in August, 1906, the first man in history to have conquered this tragic passage.

On September 3, 1986 the captain of our ship, the World Discoverer, gathered all the passengers together in the main salon and announced that we must remain anchored here at Beechey Island in Lancaster Sound because the Ottawa Ice Command radioed our ship that thick ice is blocking our passage through Prince Regent Inlet and Bellot Strait. Also, Peel Sound may also be iced in. Peel Sound was the route used by Amundsen.

The ice breakers maintained by the Canadian Coast Guard stood by us all day—also waiting for the decision on the condition of the ice in Peel Sound. Peel Sound, 200 miles south of us, is a narrow passage through which we must pass or turn back towards Greenland, Labrador and the Atlantic Ocean. I can well understand why only 36 vessels have ever made this journey and why even today with all our technology, the ice has still not been conquered. Although man has been in the Arctic for centuries, the moon's surface has been more accurately charted than the geography of the Northwest Passage.

There remained one other alternative passage and that's through the Prince Regent Inlet.

There was on board our vessel a former sea captain who is an expert ice master. His name is Tom Pullen and his job was to advise the captain of the ship on all matters concerning the ice. The decision was made not

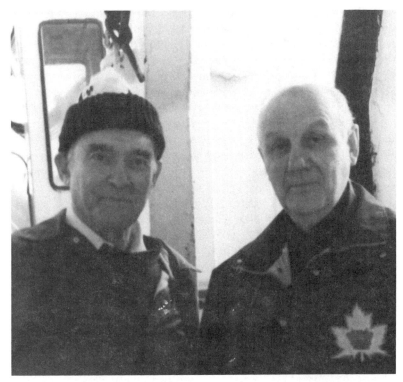

The author with Tom Pullen, the expert ice master whose decision regarding the navigability of the ice was final.

to go through Peel Sound; the ice was too thick. We were in the Prince Regent Inlet. Ice totally surrounded us and I could hear it crunching against the side of the ship as it wriggled its way through this endless white, irregular forest of snow-covered ice as far as the eye could see. If I were in Antarctica I would be under constant fear of being locked in the ice for the coming winter. But we all knew the Canadian ice breakers and reconnaissance planes were keeping an eye on our progress. Here in the North rescue is always at hand, but not so in Antarctica.

Flying above and around the ship are a variety of birds which usually pay us visits, or sit on the ice and stare at us. Among the birds we have seen so far are ravens, parasitic jaegers, arctic terns, fulmans, snow buntings, rock ptarmigans, and black-legged kittiwakes.

These fancy names came from several bird watchers who are always with high powered binoculars hanging around their necks.

The polar ice that I keep referring to has an interesting history. It is not like the ice cubes in our refrigerators, or like the icicles hanging off our roofs in winter. The Eskimos have fifty words for different kinds of ice. The ice floes through which this ship was zigzagging, can be made up of thousands of different kinds of ice depending on its age, shape, thickness, salinity, and snow cover. Fresh water freezes at 32 degrees Fahrenheit, sea water freezes at 28.6 degrees Fahrenheit. The more salt in the water the lower the freezing point. Fresh water entering the ocean from a river will freeze up at the river mouth before the ocean freezes. That's why Amundsen was beset in the ice at the mouth of the Mackenzie River of Alaska right after he completed the most complex portion of the Northwest Passage.

The first sign of freezing ocean water is an oily opaque appearance caused by the formation of ice spicules and thin plates of ice known as frazil crystals. These multiply giving the sea a slushy appearance. The ice then forms a thin elastic crust called ice rind and appears black or gray. As this rind thickens the motion of the sea breaks it up into separate masses. These masses begin to adhere forming a continuous sheet known as young ice, which becomes 3 to 4 inches thick in the first 24 hours. By the end of an Arctic winter this young ice may be as thick as 4 to 5 feet.

Half of this winter ice disappears during the short Arctic summer. As it melts the sea around the ice floe becomes covered with a thin layer of fresh water which seeps under the ice and freezes on to the underside while the top of the floe is melting. A large ice floe that survives the summer contains a greater portion of fresh water than it had the preceding winter. As ice loses its salt or salinity, it becomes harder and changes color from green to pale blue and later to bright blue. Finally sea ice becomes polar ice which is made up of almost entirely fresh water and becomes as hard as steel. An ice floe in the Arctic can be as small as 2 or 3 feet or as wide as 6 miles. These floes often join to form ice fields that can extend for hundreds of miles.

As we sailed down the Prince Regent Inlet located between Somerset Island and the Brodeur Peninsula of Baffin Island our ship encountered an ice field that was over 100 miles long.

Yet in the heart of winter there are stretches of open water even at the North Pole, because sea ice is continually driven by wind and tide. When polar floes meet gently they ride up on each other. But when the wind rises, the floes crash into each other, producing instant hummocks of ice. These ridges or hummocks can be as high as 20 to 30 feet. Ice breakers try to zigzag around these high hummocks rather than hit them head on which is what our ship was doing.

The bow of our ship shuddered as it struck the bigger floes, then the shock wave travelled the length of the ship. Just before plowing into these giant floes our ship would reverse engines, the racket of which could be heard on all the decks. Reversing the engines slowed the ship so it would not crash into the ice, but would gently split it and create a pathway for the length of the ship to pass through.

The magnificent, extremely beautiful ocean highway known as the Northwest Passage is seldom less than 50 miles wide and consists, not of one route, but of alternate routes, one or two of which are usually blocked by ice in any month of the year. The actual charting of these routes, which wind their way through multiple islands covered by perpetual ice and snow, was not completed until after World War II when aerial reconnaissance completed the charting.

Our voyage had the advantage of Canadian aerial reconnaissance as well as a stand-by ice breaker to guide us through one of the seven routes not totally choked by ice. The early explorers like Baffin, Parry, Franklin, and Amundsen never enjoyed this modern luxury.

Extreme cold is the greatest barrier to industrial development in the Arctic. At sub-zero temperatures engines have to be thawed out by blow torches. Water condenses and freezes in the fuel lines of aircraft and bulldozers. Even antifreeze turns to slush. Rubber tires split open. The blades of an ax must be warmed before it is used or it will splinter like glass. A sharply struck nail slivers into fragments. The moisture on a match head freezes. So does ink in a fountain pen. Camera shutters jam as mine did on one occasion when trying to photograph a polar bear eating a seal, and film cracks. For human protection from the cold nothing is as efficient as the Eskimo's polar bear or caribou parka, bear skin pants and boots. Polar explorers seldom grow beards since exhaled breath condenses in a beard and freezes into a mask of ice.

On Thursday, September 4, 1986, our ship, the World Discoverer, took the entire day to traverse Prince Regent Inlet to the entrance of Bellot Strait. The ship inched along, zigzagged, sped up, slowed down, backed up, all because of this ubiquitous ice which dogged our path. The sea was so cold that should anyone fall overboard he would be unconscious within two minutes due to loss of body heat. How efficiently insulated is our companion, the polar bear, who lives in this water and on the ice without even boots for his paws. At times the ship went slower than a person walking so as not to cause the sharp ice to punch a hole in the sides of our ship, or break a blade on our propellers. The bow or front of the ship was doubly reinforced to strike the ice, but it was not built as a real ice breaker. The captain, therefore, was taking no chances by ramming into the ice. He would come up to it, touch it gently, then rev up the engines and split it. I could hear the ice crunching, rumbling and scratching and clawing at the sides of the ship as we inched our way down 100 miles of this beautiful but treacherous icy, frozen, Arctic sea.

I think at times that the excitement of this trip is not only the indescribable beauty, serenity, seclusion and loneliness of the sullen brooding sky and sea, but also the ever present danger that you sense lurking in the background, but never give voice to with fellow passengers.

We anchored at the southern tip of Somerset Island, at the entrance to the 18-mile Bellot Strait.

By zodiac we landed on Somerset Island and explored an old Hudson's Bay Company outpost known as Fort Ross which was abandoned many years ago. An old stuffed chair in the living quarters appeared to have been ripped apart by a polar bear. One of the ship's officers was sent out by zodiac before the passengers to locate himself on top of one of the snowy barren hills. He sat there with a high powered telescopic rifle loaded with 38 magnum bullets in the event a polar bear got near one of the ship's passengers. Polar bears are one of the dangers which lurk in the Arctic. Since he has no predators, he is the supreme predator of the Arctic, the king of this bleak domain, as the tiger is the king of the jungle.

The word Arctic comes from the Greek word ARKTOS which means bear. It refers to any area in the far north without trees and characterized by permafrost and cold. The Arctic Ocean is five times as large as the Mediterranean Sea. A layer of the ice from one to 10 feet unites three of the world's six continents, making it possible for polar bears to circle the globe with only an occasional swim. Winds keep the polar ice pack in almost constant motion in a giant, clockwise spiral. Ice movement has been clocked at 50 miles a day. This constant ice drift means that a polar bear, in order to remain in a favorite seal rich area must compensate for the drifting ice by travelling steadily in the opposite direction.

No polar bear can survive for long away from the ice of the Arctic Ocean. Ice is the bears hunting platform, and away from it they are restless and nervous. Polar bears who have been tagged with radio transmitters have moved between Alaska, Canada and Siberia, but generally they tend to remain in the areas where they were born.

There are no polar bears in Antarctica; it is too cold.

In 1937, the Hudson's Bay Co. established an outpost at Ft. Ross as a

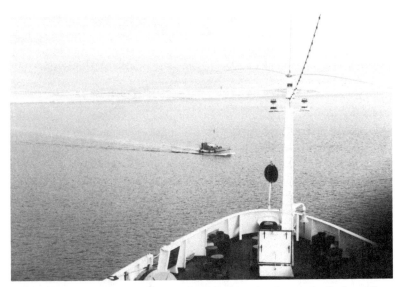

Robert Cooper's small vessel attempting to follow our ship through the Northwest Passage. The Canadian Coast Guard forbade him to do this.

trading center for buying furs from Eskimos. The Eskimos moved on to better hunting grounds and the Hudson's Bay Company's living quarters for the manager was abandoned in 1947.

A small boat was anchored in the cove at Ft. Ross, owned by a Robert Cooper who had sailed it around the world and was now preparing to sail it through one of the seven alternative routes of the Northwest Passage. Our ship gave him some food, a parka, and some fuel. He was travelling alone and upon sighting our ship hoped to follow us through the passage. The coast guard ice breaker told him not to since there was doubt that we could get through and he might be frozen in the ice. He remained behind in the cove and understood that he might have to winter over at this Hudson's Bay abandoned house till next summer since there was no exit for him. I felt very lonely for him as our ship sailed through Bellot Strait and saw him disappear as a small dot in the frozen distant landscape.

The Bellot Strait was ice-free since the current running through it flows at 8 miles an hour, faster than our ship was sailing, and the fast current prevented the water from freezing.

When we traversed the 18-mile strait the ice breaker was waiting for us at the ice-bound Peel Sound. This ice was one continuous, solid, ice desert, with no breaks. We could have walked on it. We followed the ice

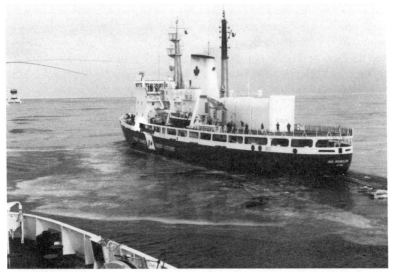

The Canadian Coast Guard ice breaker, Des Groseillers guides our ship through newly forming ice in the Northwest Passage.

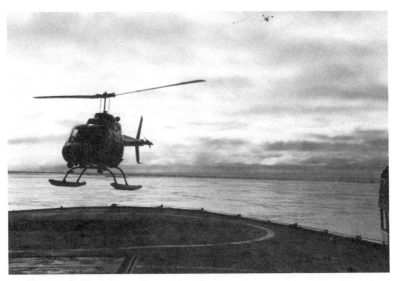

Helicopter for ice reconnaissance landing on deck of the Canadian Ice breaker. Note only two blades so that the helicopter can be stored in a narrow hanger on deck.

breaker known as the Pierre Ratison for several miles at about a mile an hour, and the helicopter reconnaissance radioed us that the thick ice extended for 150 miles all the way to King William Island and Gjoa Haven. The Canadian ice breaker had the authority to tell us to turn back or continue on. Since the ice breaker could hardly crack the ice itself, and it was getting thicker and thicker, he commanded us to turn back. As a result our ship joined the 500-year history of failures to sail the Northwest Passage. The number of successes still remain at 36. When Amundsen sailed it in 1906 he too was beset by the ice, but he wintered over at Gjoa Haven and waited a year for the ice to thaw sufficiently for him to continue.

An entire day was spent turning around and sailing back up Prince Regent Inlet toward Lancaster Sound and Fort Ross. We saw Robert Cooper's boat still anchored where we left him. He will soon have to endure three months of total darkness. His biggest danger besides 60° below zero temperatures during the long Arctic night is invasion by polar bears who will detect the odor of his cooking. The polar bear can detect the smell of bacon cooking from 15 miles away. One blow of his paw could knock down the tiny Hudson's Bay house which Cooper expects to occupy. The captain of our ship invited him aboard to deliver him back to civilization. He refused to abandon his ship. He has a wife and a new-born child in London and I fear they will never see him again.

When we had almost reached the exit of the Prince Regent Inlet we were following a new coast guard ice breaker named Des Groseilliers. Several miles before reaching Lancaster Sound, the eastern portion of Parry Channel, the ice breaker stopped. We tied up beside it and got an infusion of diesel fuel. The captain invited us aboard to visit his ship, and our ship played host to his 60-man crew.

The ice breaker had a luxurious interior, plus a two-bladed helicopter garage right on the deck.

I was interested in the engine room since an ice breaker is all engine with a ship built around it. The engines consisted of six diesels which generated 870 volts of alternating current electricity.

This voltage was fed into giant, solid-state rectifiers which converted the A.C. to 870 volts D.C. with a maximum of 6787 amperes. The D.C. voltage was used to energize the two electric motors, the shafts of which drove the two propellers made of steel so strong it was capable of grinding up ice as efficiently as kitchen mixmasters.

The chief engineer on the ice breaker was a beautiful, young lady, aged 32, who was in charge of all the diesels and generators.

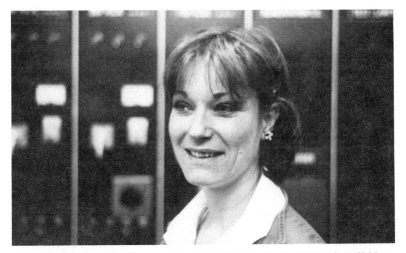

The only female among 62 men on board the Canadian ice breaker is a beautiful brunette who is the chief engineer in charge of the diesel generators and the entire engine room.

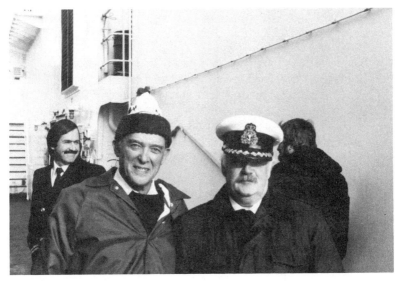

The author, left, and the Captain of the Des Groseillers ice breaker, standing next to the on-deck hangar for the helicopter.

The captain of the ice breaker was kind enough to have his picture taken with me next to him.

The major problem with attempting the Northwest Passage is, of course, ice. A ship can proceed down an inlet (there are seven possible ways to get through) but 20 miles down the inlet the ship can be faced with an insurmountable ice barrier. The ship must turn around if it can, go back, and try another route that may also be iced in. This is what happened for 500 years.

In 1968, the Humble Oil and Atlantic Richfield Oil Companies found one of the largest oil fields in the world on the North coast of Alaska at Prudhoe Bay near Point Barrow, right on the Arctic Ocean which was mostly frozen in winter and at times during the three months of summer. Before they built the Alaska Pipe Line which brought the oil to Valdez, Alaska's southern warm water port, they thought of shipping it by tanker through the Northwest Passage. This, they thought, was a viable alternative since a pipe line across Alaska would require pumping the oil from Point Barrow into a tanker at Valdez, sailing the oil to the Isthmus of Panama, then they would need another pipe line next to the Panama Canal to carry the oil across Panama and then pump it again into oil tankers on the Atlantic side of the canal since oil tankers are too big for the Panama Canal itself. It would then be shipped to the U.S. east coast, a long expensive journey. They could save one million dollars a day by, somehow, opening the Northwest Passage, the gateway to Europe and the U.S. industrial, east coast.

The oil companies acquired the largest oil tanker in the world, The Manhattan, and converted it into an experimental ice breaker with the objective of making a trial run through the Northwest Passage. It had a prow of two-inch-thick, tensile steel. A second steel hull was built around the engine room. The propellers, 25 feet in diameter were made of a special nickel, bronze, aluminum alloy. It had a helicopter pad. It had a steel 16-foot-high ice belt, 8 feet thick capable of withstanding the hardest ice. The ship was as long as the Empire State Building, 1005 feet.

It had engines that developed the power of 43,000 horses going forward and only 15,000 in reverse. It had radio communication 500 times more powerful than any other ship afloat. This was an experimental ship designed as a prototype for future tankers that could conquer the ice. The ship had electronic sensors to record measurements of ice strain at 400 points around the ship and temperature at 50 other locations and television cameras to transmit pictures showing how the ice broke around the bow and the stern. This information was fed into computers which were to be used later to design oil tankers if this one developed flaws and failed to traverse the Northwest Passage.

The giant tanker set sail from the shipbuilding yard in Chester, Pennsylvania, and, after sailing past Nova Scotia, up the Davis Strait bordering the coast of Greenland, it entered the Northwest Passage at Lancaster Sound and sailed west past all of the inlets and sounds that my ship had traversed. They stopped at Beechey Island as I did, passed Resolute where my plane landed from Edmonton and tried to buck the ice in McClure Strait. They had helicopters for reconnaissance plus Canadian ice breakers to assist them. They rammed the ice hoping to crack it, but the ship just slipped up on the 20 foot thick ice and there they were stuck and could not work the giant tanker loose.

On board were newspaper men, CBS and Canadian television crews, and a host of foreign correspondents who were recording this great historic event—an oil tanker attempting the Northwest Passage.

On board was Captain Tom Pullen who was also on board my ship. He is an ice master who advised our captain on decisions regarding the ice. They were stuck in the ice. The passengers, many of whom were officials of Exxon and Humble Oil Co., all got off the ship to walk around on the ice. A lookout kept watch for polar bears. They finally backed the Manhattan out after one of the small Canadian ice breakers cut out a section of ice at the stern of the ship.

The ship had to turn around and attempt one of the alternate routes which was the Prince of Wales Strait.

They finally made a successful passage and took on a symbolic barrel of oil at Point Barrow, Alaska. Then they returned successfully through the Northwest Passage and out into the Atlantic Ocean and ended the journey in New York Harbor in 1969.

Because of the unpredictability of the ice, the problem of an oil spill which would contaminate the passage and result in the death of seals which polar bears feed on, plus the enormous cost of tanker ice breakers, which, without an accompanying second ice breaker, could not be relied upon, the idea of using tankers died at birth. The six-billion-dollar, Alaska oil pipe line was constructed instead. The mission of the Manhattan tanker went into the history books as another attempt to conquer that ice giant of the North that was only partially successful.

The finale to this story is this. The oil companies were convinced in advance on the superiority of the Alaska pipe line since most of the oil is consumed on the west coast of the United States anyway. The Alaskan fields produce a million barrels of oil a day. But this country needs 18 million barrels of oil a day to fuel our automobiles and factories. The 17 million extra barrels come from the middle east, Kuwait, Iraq, Iran, Saudi-Arabia, Nigeria, and Venezuela, most of which, if they would ever stop killing each other, could strangle the U.S., Europe and Japan who are totally dependent on them.

The purpose of this Manhattan tanker project was a lobbying project to get Congress to okay the Alaska pipe line. The oil companies knew they couldn't get oil into tankers off the Alaska coast since the water in the Beaufort sea is only 30 feet deep as far out as 100 miles, which is not deep enough for these giant oil tankers to dock in. They had to prove to the Congressmen that going through the ice was impractical. The several million they spent rebuilding the Manhattan was simply lobbying money to get Congress to approve construction of the Alaskan pipe line. All is not as simple as it appears.

THE NORTH MAGNETIC POLE

The north magnetic pole is where we boarded this ship at Resolute. The north geographic pole is farther north. The magnetic pole is the point to which compasses point north. At this position, right at the north magnetic pole, compasses go wild; they keep spinning and do not know in which direction to stop since almost every point is south from here. The ship depends on satellite and inertial guidance for direction and also employs a gyroscopic compass.

The interesting aspect of this north magnetic pole is that it keeps moving every 24 hours in an elliptical path that may cover over 100 miles. Once again it was that great explorer Amundsen who defined the north magnetic pole in 1904 when his vessel, the Gjoa was beset in the ice at Gjoa Haven during his journey through the Northwest Passage. For 23 months he recorded the position of the pole every day. The movement of the pole is caused by the movement of the magnetic field in the center of the earth. Its position is also altered by the aurora borealis, solar winds, and destruction of portions of the Van Allen Belt when atomic explosions occur.

When there was no longer any ice blocking our progress, we turned back and sailed north off the east coast of Devon Island out in Baffin Bay. We headed toward Ellesmere Island and several Eskimo outposts near the shore. The sea was sprinkled with white caps since there was no ice in sight to tame the waves. Icebergs, however, were evident.

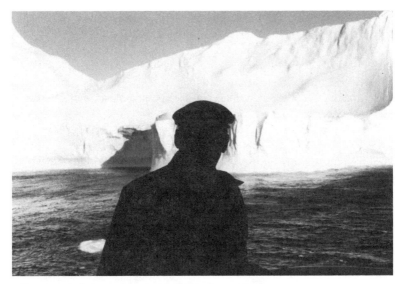

Enormous icebergs are prevalent in the Northwest Passage.

We sailed up Baffin Bay, through Smith Sound into Kane Basin. Only 21 miles separate Ellesmere Island (Canada) from Greenland. We reached to within a few miles of 80° latitude—only 600 miles from the geographic North Pole. The sea exhibited a greasy gray appearance indicating the beginning of new winter ice which would within a few weeks lock this land into a vise-like, impenetrable, frozen grip. We circled around an enormous iceberg at least 12 stories high and one city block long. Cameras were clicking from every open area and window of the ship. Much of Baffin Bay is at present ice-free except for numerous icebergs. There is a peculiar warming geography in this area that prevents the sea from freezing to a great depth. The inlets and sounds branching off Baffin Bay were all frozen as if winter was already there.

There is a small Eskimo settlement on the northwest coast of Greenland known as Etah, right on the northwest edge of Smith Sound. We attempted a landing but the sea was so rough the zodiaks had to turn back. Despite 16 pieces of clothing which included three pairs of socks in knee-high rubber boots, I was still cold, the temperature being far below zero. The Eskimo families who live on Etah live there by hunting for fish, birds, caribou, polar bears and seals. They have no contact with civilization, no electricity, no radio, no TV, no telephone. They live in this deep freeze which is below zero in summer, as well as winter.

This Etah outpost was visited by most of the Arctic explorers, since it is on a direct route to the North Pole. Admiral Perry stopped here as well as other polar explorers. This Etah is an important historic center. Admiral Perry's wife had a baby here in the early 1900's. There is evidence that this area was occupied by humans as long as 4000 years ago.

Several days later the ship docked at the southernmost tip of Ellesmere Island, located on the Jones Sound.

Everyone piled into zodiacs to explore an Eskimo village known as Grise Fiord.

This village is located on a flat, pebbly beach, about three blocks in depth with mountains that rise straight up. There was a wooden church, a new school, a hospital with an R.N. in charge. All these buildings rested on posts with a three-to-four foot space under the building to prevent the permafrost from melting.

The Eskimos live by hunting seals, fox, caribou, and polar bears. The skins of these animals are stretched in front of their houses to dry and are later sold.

The Canadian Government it seems, has a big heart in supporting the Eskimos. They use skidoos instead of dog sleds to transport them over the mountains which surround them. The nurse is an R.N. from Canada. She knows how to extract a tooth, how to place a filling and how to inject novocain to make fillings or extractions pain-free.

This Eskimo community at *Grise Fiord,* 700 miles north of the Arctic Circle is typical of many Eskimo outposts throughout the high Arctic. The population is almost 110. There are several white souls here who run the school which goes to 8th grade. There is a fish scientist who spends time here with his wife. They live in a 12 × 16 one-story box and are conducting ice and animal migration studies for the Canadian Government.

The invasion of the remote Eskimo outposts by white Canadians known as "southerners" has posed numbers of problems for the Eskimo and his way of life. The situation is partly similar to the encirclement of our Indian reservations in Arizona and New Mexico.

Eskimos are the epitome of friendliness and are self-sufficient. They do not depend on outsiders. They are sharing and most cooperative. The big general store is cooperatively owned. It is not a Hudson's Bay Company that attempts to buy their seal and bear skins for pennies and resell them for hundreds of dollars. If a family has four children and a fifth comes along, which is too much for the mother, the next door neighbor with only two children will rear the child. All the Eskimos are an extended family. They live by hunting and fishing, and the catch of seal or fish is shared among them.

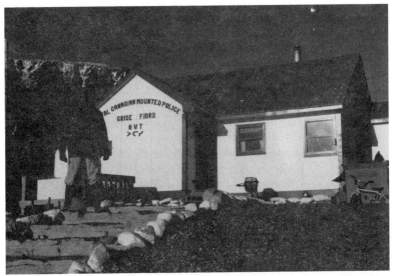

The Police station at Grise Fiord, an Eskimo outpost located at the southern tip of Ellesmere Island.

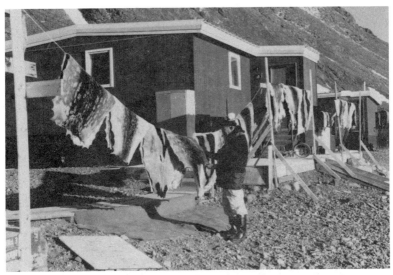

Eskimos live by hunting animals. The skins are stretched in front of their cabins to dry and are later sold.

An Eskimo can eat five or six pounds of seal or caribou meat at a single meal. One husky dog requires as much food as a man. As winter approaches the high Arctic most of the birds head south. Only the raven, the snowy owl, the ptarmigan and the gerfalcon remain. The birds adopt a white coloring as camouflage against predators. Only the raven remains glossy black in a world of whiteness.

The seasonal activities and migration of animals has a powerful effect on Eskimo life. The establishment of Grise Fiord came about because of the richness of the sea with seals and fish at this particular location.

Then the "southerners" came in and introduced the rifle to kill caribou and bears. Once the convenience of a rifle was demonstrated there was no going back to the harpoon. Once the white man showed the Eskimos the simplicity and permanence of house building there was no going back to caribou-skin tents and igloos. And with the introduction of motorized sleds known as skidoos, the dog-team sled became obsolete. Now they have, not black and white TV, but color. Microwave ovens are in every shack.

The age of death 22 years ago was 36. Today Eskimos live an average of 50 years.

Deafness has become a major environmental problem due to sitting over the loud motor of the skidoos when they set out to hunt. The loudness has caused deafness.

Alcohol and drugs, another white man importation, is also taking its toll.

Tooth decay is rampant and the cause can be seen in the cooperative general store where candy bins, cake, ice cream, wheaties and cocoa puffs, all made with sugar and, of course, the ubiquitous Coca Cola an I Pepsi.

The Eskimos are trying to synthesize their culture with that of the white man's convenience. The Eskimos are not against science, but they want to retain their hunting-for-food culture and all the customs that accompany it.

This Grise Fiord is so far north that it is locked in by ice for nine months of the year, three months of which are in total darkness. I spoke to an unemployed 20-year-old, male Eskimo. "Since you cannot find work here would you consider going South into Canada for employment?" He wouldn't hear of it. This was his home.

The Canadian Government is attempting to place restrictions on the number of seals, bears, white fox, and caribou they can kill. The Eskimo resents the white man's intrusion into his food supply.

The Eskimo is content with his culture but he is inquisitive as to why birds breed in the Arctic then fly south; and why whales breed up here then swim to the other side of the world. They say to the white man, go ahead with your scientific investigations, but give us dollars and we will run our own communities, we will develop our own policies and laws. Canada is reluctant to do this.

The high Arctic which comprises a large area known as N.W.T. or North West Territories is the home of the Eskimos. They compromise one-third of the people who live there. The Eskimo population in the N.W.T. is estimated at 45,000. They call themselves not the disadvantaged 3rd world, but the 4th world. The 3rd world was colonized by war, but not the Eskimo. They believe animals are here to be hunted for food, and not conserved and restricted as is the southern belief. Wildlife is the economic base of the Eskimo community. They do not like to work in mines because they cannot see the sun. And when the goose migration starts in its season the Eskimo must hunt.

The Canadian Parliament has two Eskimos, one from the eastern and one from the western section of the N.W.T. The N.W.T. is now an independent state in Canada, like Alberta, or Quebec, similar to the relationship that California or Maryland has to the U.S. Federal Government.

I visited another Eskimo settlement located at the Clyde Inlet, a fiord on the east coast of Baffin Island, still in the high Arctic 250 miles north of the Arctic Circle.

There is a large Eskimo outpost known as the Clyde River Village consisting of 500 Eskimos and 22 whites. The whites run the Hudson's Bay Co. community store. They are teachers in a newly constructed school with grades from 1 through 10. There is one policeman, a member of the RCMP—The Royal Canadian Mounted Police.

The Eskimos live in wooden houses of varying colors, have skidoos, bicycles, refrigerators, TV sets, microwave ovens and other modern conveniences. The streets are not paved and everyone wears rubber boots.

Our ship was the first ship to visit this outpost in half a year. School was dismissed so that the children could see the parka-clad passengers come ashore in zodiaks. Three weeks previously the inlet was a mass of impenetrable ice. On this day it was ice free. The ice did not melt, it was simply blown out into Baffin Bay. The ice in the high Arctic is extremely unpredictable.

I visited the Hudson's Bay general store and bought post cards. Prices of food were exorbitant. A head of lettuce was $3.25, milk was $3.19 a quart, one green pepper, $1.95.

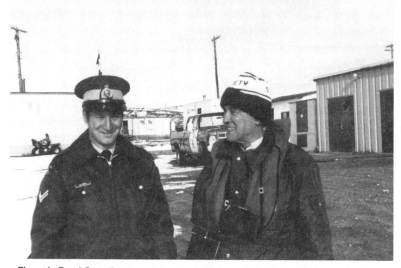

The only Royal Canadian mounted policeman at the Clyde River Eskimo outpost on the east coast of Baffin Island. He keeps order among 500 Eskimos and 22 whites. He does not appear as warmly dressed as the author.

Inquiries revealed the following: Most of the Eskimos are unemployed and receive from the NWT (Northwest Territory) government and from the federal Canadian Government a welfare check every two weeks. The NWT check goes directly to the Hudson's Bay General Store and they can purchase food against this check. The other check goes directly to the Eskimo. The total income for a husband, wife and one child is about $1,000 a month—when he does *not work*. When he works his income as a truck driver emptying septic tanks could be as high as $35,000 a year.

The geographic setting for this Clyde River Village is quite beautiful. The inlet from Baffin Bay which is several miles long ends in a round, dead-end pouch, several miles across, surrounded by ice and snow-covered hills. On the top of one of the hills is a large, white satellite dish which makes direct-dialing telephone communication with the rest of the world a reality, plus TV reception. There is a landing strip for propeller type planes, but not for jets.

The Eskimo still hunts for seal, caribou, fox and wolves. I bought a wolf skin right off the wall of an Eskimo's house for $10.00. He showed me the inside of his refrigerator. It was empty except for a big chunk of frozen seal meat that his next door neighbor gave him. The Eskimos share

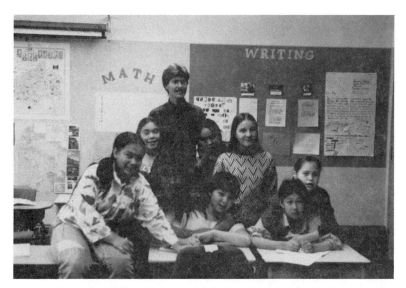

A Canadian teacher in the school at the Clyde River Eskimo outpost on Baffin Island.

everything with neighbors that lack things such as meat. They eat the seal raw. Sometimes they make a soup of pieces of it.

The school building is only two years old. The first language is Inuktitut. The second language is English. The Canadian teachers (whites) truly earn their pay trying to make children learn mathematical concepts in their second language, since the white teacher cannot communicate in Inuktitut, the Eskimo language.

In this community I once again examined teeth. There is much decay.

All medical and dental services are free. This immense area known as the NWT is predominantly Eskimo since few white people would ever consider living in a perpetual deep freeze where total darkness exists for 3 months of the year with an average temperature of 40 to 60 degrees below zero.

The Canadian Government flies soldiers to these Eskimo outposts to train unemployed and other volunteer Eskimos in how to handle rifles, how to march and how to obey military commands. I questioned an army captain as to why Canada undertakes this military expenditure. "Just to make the Eskimos understand the existence of a military presence in the high Arctic," he said.

Outside the large school building are playgrounds and in the schools are bulletin boards in all the hallways. On the bulletin boards are placards

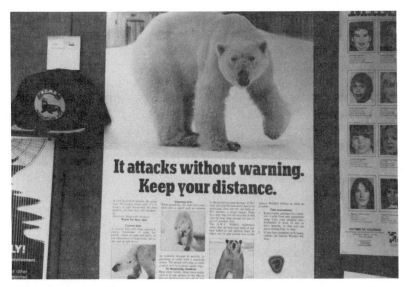

Polar Bears are a constant threat to Eskimos. Placards on the school bulletin boards alert children to this menace. To the right are faces of children who have been attacked or killed by Polar Bears.

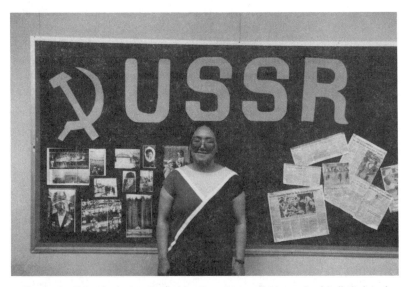

The Soviet Union is depicted as a friendly nation on Eskimo school bulletin boards. There is an exchange program between Soviet and Canadian Eskimos.

warning what to do if one encounters a polar bear. There are also displays of the Soviet hammer and sickle, with newspaper articles and headlines depicting life in the U.S.S.R. as being very friendly and neighborly. There is an exchange program between Soviet Eskimos and Canadian Eskimos, all in the interest of establishing friendship between the two countries. This is something that Ronald Reagan and his followers have yet to learn. Sexual relations between the teenagers is freer than in the U.S. If they decide to live together, the boy moves into the girl's house. Marriage may or may not occur.

The entire village is nestled on the permafrost next to the water, surrounded by the low, snow-covered hills. Everyone knows everyone else. The Eskimos are like one big, interrelated family, and they care for one another.

In another Eskimo outpost known as Pangnirtung, located in a fiord at the northern end of Cumberland Sound, an offshoot of Baffin Bay, there live one thousand Eskimos and 20 white Canadians. There are two Royal Canadian Mounted Police who are kept busy tracking house robberies which number about two a day. The thieves are Eskimo teenagers who steal chocolate cookies and cans of Del Monte peaches or pears. They never take VCR's or TV sets, just sweets. There are two supermarkets, one a cooperative and the other a Hudson's Bay Company. This settlement is "dry" meaning no alcohol can be sold or exist in any household. The mounted policeman told me the theft of sweets and canned fruits was to make illegal alcohol.

To appreciate where and how these communities thrive one must sail from the open sea (Baffin Bay) turn into a fiord and sail for miles up this fiord. Off in the distance, sitting in a curved arm of the fiord, the outpost soon appears. Small, multicolored little boxes called houses, are nestled on a flat pebbled area at the foot of a snow-capped mountain. As the ship comes closer the first objects that stand out are the huge white, concave, microwave discs aimed at the satellite in the sky for telephone and TV reception. The next large object is the depot of multistoried fuel tanks and diesel sheds for generating electricity. These outposts are isolated, and seemingly cut off from civilization. They would be if not for telephone, TV and radio reception. Our ship, the World Discoverer, was the first passenger vessel to ever visit this community. They usually see only three freight vessels a year: one carries the merchandise and food to supply the Hudson's Bay Co. supermarket. The next vessel is a fuel ship to fill their diesel tanks for generating electricity, and to supply gasoline for their Skidoos. The third vessel brings lumber, plumbing supplies, toilet paper,

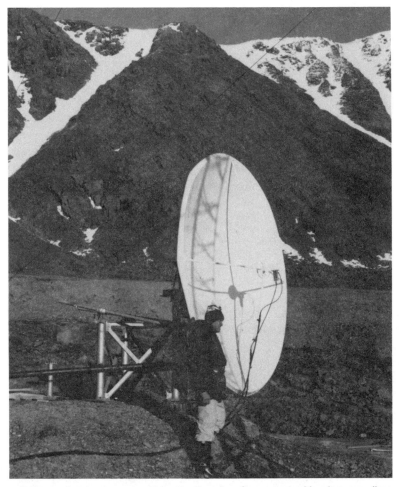

Eskimo outposts are equipped by the Canadian Government with microwave discs aimed at the satellite in the sky for telephone and TV reception.

flour and all the other supplies needed in the Eskimo-operated cooperative general store.

The inhabitants knew several days in advance by telex and radio that the first passenger ship ever to sail to this lonely forsaken place would arrive on Sunday, September 14th. The entire Eskimo population was lined up on the shore to greet these red-parka-clad visitors with rubber boots from another planet. What a reception it was! They had trucks and automobiles waiting and ready to transport us from the rubber zodiaks on the pebbly

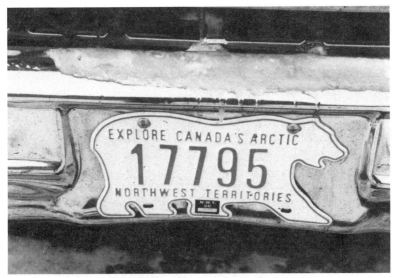

License plates are in the shape of a Polar Bear in the Canadian High Arctic.

beach up to their community. Our ship, meanwhile, transported the excited Eskimos in the zodiaks back to our big ship anchored three miles out in the fiord. The water at the beach was too shallow for our big ship. Kindness and hospitality of such dimension are very seldomly experienced. The school teachers and senior students were our guides through the six-block-long community.

The houses, of course, were on stilts so as not to affect the permafrost. And each house had a telephone and all the conveniences known only in the "south" which meant Canadian civilization 1,000 miles away. The school principal, teachers, policeman, communication experts, and managers of all stores, weaving factory and print shops were all white. Eskimos were definitely not running the Pangnirtung outpost. Autos have Canadian license plates in the shape of a polar bear. Septic tanks are emptied periodically.

There were several dog teams that pulled sleds when the Eskimos went out on a seal or caribou hunt. The Eskimos eat the seal raw. Seal meat is a complete food when eaten uncooked. They all say the taste is delicious. When uncooked it has all the vitamins and minerals one needs to maintain good health in addition to protein and fat which metabolize to carbohydrate. The foods they sell in the Hudson's Bay Co. are poison to these seal and caribou eaters. Yet they'll buy this junk food when seal meat is not available.

The young, unmarried girls get pregnant about as often as Baltimore's disadvantaged population, but abortions are not performed. There's always some family that will raise the child since the mother may be in the 9th or 10th grade. Since the Eskimos are one large extended family, there's no stigma to pregnancy out of wedlock. Marriages may occur after the girl shows evidence of being pregnant. Three weeks prior to our arrival an Eskimo killed his wife and child, then shot himself. Reasons were unknown. The house they lived in is now empty and no Eskimo will live there. So the home remains empty despite a shortage of homes.

Eskimo settlements in the high arctic are based on an economy consisting of hunting whales, seals, caribou and polar bears. These animals meet the three essentials to human life: food, clothing and shelter. Food comes from the meat. Spoilage does not occur since the entire Arctic is one big refrigerator summer and winter. Clothing from caribou skin is superior to wool or any synthetic fiber man could ever devise. Shelter comes from caribou skins sewn together and fashioned into a tent supported by walrus tusks or whale bones. Oil for the shelter comes from rendering caribou and seal fat. Igloos are temporary houses built on the ice when the family goes on a hunt that could last for a week or more. So it's quite obvious that Eskimos are a self sufficient people.

Eskimos people the Arctic of Canada, Greenland, Finland and the northern USSR. They migrated from Siberia across the Bering Strait over 4,000 years ago as determined by carbon dating of their excavated tools.

The Eskimos believed animals had souls, and thanked the slaughtered animals, taking pains to explain they had killed to provide for life's needs. Treated with so much respect, they reasoned, the souls would be placated, and future reincarnations would be more inclined to give themselves up to hunters. Contemptuous treatment would surely provoke their god Sedna to withhold her bounty.

Respect for the slaughtered seal or polar bear was a specific act. This consisted of washing the dead animal's mouth with fresh water. They still use kayaks for water transportation.

In 1719 two Dutchmen sailing up the west coast of Greenland stumbled into a multimillion dollar breeding area for whales. Our ship sailed right through this area of the Baffin Bay. For the next 300 years whalers from Germany, England, Scotland, Holland and New England killed practically every whale in Baffin Bay. Whales meant big cash fortunes for their oil and by-products such as soap, cosmetics, pharmaceuticals, and whalebones for umbrella ribs, corset stays, skirt hoops and typewriter springs.

When an Eskimo caught a whale he could exchange it for tea, flour, steel needles, scissors, wooden boats, (there being no trees in the Arctic.) They paid the price for trading and social mixing with the traders who infused into their bodies syphilis, gonorrhea, tuberculosis, mumps and measles. Eskimos were never infected by these plagues and therefore had no immunity against the outbreak of these diseases.

When they had guns with which to shoot seals and caribou, they had to have trading posts to buy bullets which could only be gotten from European traders. There was simply no going back to the spear or hand-held harpoon.

When whales became scarce due to the unrestricted wholesale slaughter by Europeans, the trading posts were shut down and abandoned like the post at Fort Ross where we sailed away from the young explorer and his boat at the Bellot Strait.

The first trading posts in the Canadian High Arctic were established by the Hudson's Bay Company which was a corporate empire that owned or administered half of Canada. They set up trading posts in almost every Eskimo community that I visited on this polar expedition including the Clyde River post, the Pangnirtung post, the abandoned Ft. Ross post at Bellot Strait, the Grise Fiord post and others. The Eskimos gave a name to the HBC and called it "Here Before Christ".

Anglican church missionaries followed quickly behind the HBC establishments, built churches, and in no time had the Eskimos converted to Christianity. Soon the RCMP (Royal Canadian Mounted Police) followed and established a police station at the Clyde River community in 1922. Later there was RCMP in all the large settlements. They began recording deaths, marriages, delivering mail and became enforcers of Canadian law.

During the Cold War with Russia after World War II the United States began construction of the DEW (Distant Early Warning) line which was a series of microwave, big concave dishes and immense grids, high up on the mountain tops, all along the Arctic Circle from Alaska to the Canadian High Arctic and across Greenland. I saw one of these ridiculous stations at Cape Dyer, high on a rocky mountain, which was visible from Baffin Bay. This DEW line was to give the U.S. three minutes warning should Soviet planes fly from Russia to bomb the U.S. This was an RCA and Westinghouse bonanza that my income tax paid for. I was appalled at the wasteful impracticality of this sort of outmoded outpost since any enemy could fire missiles from submarines right off our coast. It is another example of the military industrial complex milking the average citizen for the benefit of corporate profits. Today all these Dew Line stations are obsolete or abandoned. Untold millions were squandered.

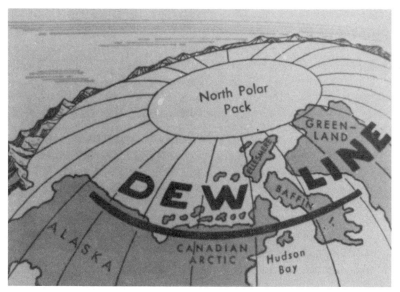

Location of the Distant Early Warning or DEW LINE radar stations established by U.S. tax dollars proved to be as wasteful an investment as Reagan's Star Wars.

Dew Line construction introduced wage labor to the Eskimo, and opened up the High Arctic to passenger expeditions. It also led to the Canadian Government's realization that fellow Canadians—i.e. Eskimos, were starving in many of their remote communities. Starvation occurred because of the sometime sudden decline in the seal and caribou populations, augmented also by the world-wide declining demand for furs.

When Eskimo famine became front page news in Ottawa, the government responded with a massive food and aid program and an intensive drive to establish medical services, schools, electric power, radio and telephone service. The Canadian Government established 13 communities with all these services in the largest island in the High Arctic, Baffin Island. We visited two of these: Clyde and Pangnirtung.

At first many of the Eskimo families were reluctant to leave their caribou tent and igloo outposts because the government centers with their HBC stores were too far removed from the best hunting grounds. With the introduction of the skidoo, the motorized sled, they could travel with great speed compared to the dog sled. This eased their concern about distance and furthered the transition from caribou camp to government-erected Eskimo towns and wooden houses.

Today in 1986 a few families are still living in caribou tents in isolated areas of the Arctic. But most prefer to reside in towns such as Clyde that have an airstrip, schools, nursing stations, churches and Hudson's Bay stores. The Eskimo still goes out on his skidoo to hunt seal and caribou which the HBC stores do not sell. The skins he tans and hangs out on his front porch to "cure".

A big sale item in the HBC store is Pampers—a disposable diaper. Most mothers carry their babies in a caribou pouch hanging off their back. The mother's back is naked, and the baby in the pouch is also naked. When the child urinates the mother can feel the warm stream on her back. She quickly snatches the naked child out of the pouch and permits him to urinate in the snow. In the general HBC stores, Pampers are stacked to the ceiling, the hottest item in the store.

Dog teams which pull Eskimo sleds over the ice are still used, but the skidoo has replaced most of them. The dogs, known as huskies, are thickly furred and usually have beautiful blue eyes.

Greenland huskies are unique to Greenland and will fight and rebel if a Canadian or Alaskan huskie is brought in to harness. When any husky has his tail up he's happy and content. When he's angry, his tail is usually down. Whenever a dog team is being established the dogs will fight among themselves to establish a leader and proper pecking order. Dog one will bite dog two and so on down the line. If this pecking order is not established, the dog team will not function and no sled will move.

The dog paws do not freeze because the soles of their feet consist of a rough horny substance, like a horse's hoof devoid of blood vessels. The dogs are taught only three commands: to stop, turn left and turn right.

The time finally arrived for the ship to turn southward in Baffin Bay and head for the David Strait and Halifax, Nova Scotia, where our journey would terminate. As the ship sailed ever south from the top of Greenland the temperature on the deck began to rise. When temperatures rise from 10 below zero to zero the difference is meaningful to an Eskimo, but it still felt cold to me. We passed the Hudson Strait and came within sight of the northern coast of Labrador which is now part of Newfoundland, even though the original Newfoundland is an island unto itself. On the map Labrador appears as the eastern coast of Quebec. Labrador has a population of 30,000 people. The Island of Newfoundland has 80,000 people. One of the main industries is harvesting Christmas trees for export to the rest of the world.

The Island of Newfoundland wants to control Labrador. They're fighting over this in the courts. It's not settled yet. But maps from as early as 1961 show Labrador in tiny letters and Newfoundland in large black type right across Labrador.

We entered the Strait of Belle Isle which divides the Island of Newfoundland from Labrador's Newfoundland and anchored a mile off the north coast of the Island of Newfoundland at the historic site known as L'Anse aux Meadows.

Boarding the zodiaks was a rough, risky jump since the Atlantic was stirred up by strong winds, probably from a hurricane that was brewing somewhere out in the Atlantic.

The zodiac sailed through a sea of four-foot waves and deposited us at an improvised dock on the shore of this remote fishing village of L'Anse aux Meadows. Scattered small houses lined the shoreline and fishermen's wives were at their windows wondering who these red parka invaders were with cameras around their necks instead of guns. I had to ask a buxom housewife who was feeding her ducks for directions to the archeological site where the Vikings landed here over 1000 years ago. She pointed to the correct direction which was about a mile down a stone road.

It is this exact spot that usurped from Columbus the title of "discoverer of America."

On a summer day 1000 years ago a vessel from Greenland docked here; its crew of 30 men stepped ashore and decided to remain here. These were the true discoverers of America 500 years before Columbus. The leader of this expedition was Leif Eriksson. The streams were packed with salmon, cod and other fish. They found grapes growing wild and named the place Vineland. The following summer Lief returned to Greenland with a shipload of lumber and grapes. The lumber was especially valuable since few trees grew in Greenland.

Lief's luck in the new country enticed others to come to Vineland. Another expedition set out with 135 men and 15 women, plus livestock. They used Lief's camp as a base and began to populate this desolate, windy, finger of Newfoundland that stuck out into the Atlantic Ocean.

These pioneers lived here long enough to build substantial houses, workshops and a small forge, where, for the first time, iron was smelted in the New World.

Archeological digs have revealed that the buildings were of the same kind as those used in Iceland and Greenland in the 10th century and numerous artifacts such as oil lamps, the fly wheel of a handheld spindle, scissors, and slag from smelting iron with a large number of iron boat nails. The archaeologists have identified this site as Norse, and these artifacts are on exhibit in a brand new museum which the Canadian Government recently built. In 1977 this site became L'ANSE AUX MEADOWS NATIONAL HISTORIC PARK, and was placed on UNESCO'S World Heritage list of Cultural and Natural sites of outstanding value. The backyards of the houses have large wire grates on which fish are dried in the sun.

In zodiaks again we took a bumpy ride to the mother ship which sailed across the Strait of Belle Isle and anchored in a beautiful calm bay known as Red Bay on the Labrador Coast of Newfoundland. The crude little dock was lined with school children. This Red Bay is a fishing village of 350 people. All the children attend one school with grades kindergarten to grade 12. The one single industry is professional fishing with huge nets. Cod is the main fish. The men catch them and the women work in the fish factory where they clean the fish, salt it, dry it and ship thousands of tons to St. Johns, Newfoundland, in trucks which board a ferry to cross the Belle Isle Strait. The dried fish are then shipped to Japan, India and to whomever has the cash to pay for it.

The people who live here all know how to ski since this entire place is frozen tight in the winter and skis are a practical method of transportation. There are two churches, two general stores and two small corner stores. The air is deliciously clean and the day I was there was unusual since the sky was the bluest blue, not gray.

The geographic position of Red Bay can only be appreciated if you look at the map. This place can only be reached by sea or air. It is absolutely cut off from the rest of the world as it nestles on the fringe of the Atlantic Ocean on the lonely, forsaken coast of cold, cold Labrador.

I queried six school children about Leif Eriksson. None of them ever heard of him. They had heard of Columbus but it wasn't clear who he was.

Their main diet is salted fish, chicken, and sometimes boiled seal meat, and of course cake, candy and Pepsi.

Labrador is an isolated, forsaken land of a hundred fiords, high, treeless mountains, locked in ice in winter, and is truly North America's last frontier. Explorer Jacques Cartier coined a phrase about Labrador to describe the austere conditions of isolation. He called it "the land God gave to Cain."

Half of Canada's entire output of iron ore comes from Labrador. There's a road that connects a line of Labrador industrial cities which are Labrador City, Wabush, Churchill Falls and Green Bay. The multiple fishing villages such as Red Bay are isolated and accessible only by sea or air.

Labrador and Newfoundland have one thing in common: that Arctic type brooding, low, sorrowful, gray sky that appears always ready to weep snow flakes.

Even bad weather has its own beauty in Newfoundland. It seems to be a land of millions of Christmas trees. The largest paper mill in the world is located in Newfoundland because of its extensive tree coverage. Paper is made by grinding up wood into a pulp, mixing it with water and pressing it between steel rollers. No chemicals are used, just woodpulp and water.

Newfoundland sticks out into the eastern Atlantic so far that one is closer to England than to Nebraska and as close to Italy as Baltimore is to California.

Water is everywhere. There are more lakes and rivers for every square mile than anywhere else in North America. It's possible to drive a hundred miles without seeing a house or meeting a living soul.

The name of this Canadian province was conferred by the explorer John Cabot who in 1497 claimed discovery of the "NEW FOUNDE LANDE" on behalf of the King of England who gave him ten pounds for his efforts.

A number of "firsts" are attributable to Newfoundland. The first transatlantic wireless signal was received by Guglielmo Marconi on Signal Hill in 1901; the departure of the first successful transatlantic airplane by Alcock and Brown in 1919; the laying of the first successful transatlantic, telegraph cable in 1866; and the first North American smallpox vaccination occurred here in 1900.

Our last port of call before ending our voyage in Halifax, was at Norris Point in Newfoundland's Bonne Bay. We were met by two school buses that drove us to the Gros Morne National Park on Newfoundland's west coast. This park is a geologist's dream. There were high mountains, bogs, sand dunes, volcanic sea-stacks, caves, and an area of archeological excavation that revealed a community of Eskimos who lived here 6000 years ago by carbon dating.

CHAPTER II

THE ANESTHESIA YEARS AT
JOHNS HOPKINS

In 1979, after retiring from dental practice at the age of 61, I was appointed to the teaching staff of the Johns Hopkins University School of Medicine in two departments: as an Assistant Professor of Anesthesia and Critical Care Medicine, and as Assistant Professor in the department of Oral and Maxillofacial Surgery.

My career prior to this appointment was detailed in a book published in 1968 entitled AS I SAW IT. I recapitulate some aspects of this earlier career by stating, in one or two paragraphs, that I was graduated from the University of Maryland School of Dentistry in 1943, and interned in dentistry at the Maryland General Hospital in Baltimore, where I was instructed (unofficially) in anesthesiology. I spent several months with Dr. John Lundy at the Mayo Clinic in Rochester, Minnesota and served a year of residency (official) in anesthesiology at the West Jersey Hospital in Camden, New Jersey. I became Chief of Anesthesiology at the South Baltimore General Hospital in 1945 and practiced medical anesthesiology for a period of 18 years, never having entered the practice of dentistry. In 1963, the anesthesia law inn Maryland changed while I was Chief of Anesthesiology at the North Charles General Hospital. Since I was a D.D.S. and not an M.D., the law said I could no longer practice medical anesthesiology but I could administer general anesthesia for dental operations. I, therefore, bought a dental practice from a retiring dentist on Mountain Road in Pasadena, Maryland, and for the first time since graduating from Dental School 20 years previously, I began to fill and extract teeth, and not too skillfully at first.

Meanwhile the law excluding me as the only dentist in Maryland from practicing medical anesthesiology, was changed. A bill was entered in the Maryland State Legislature known as the "Grandfather Bill" which permitted me to continue to practice medical anesthesiology. The bill known as H.R. 263 was passed by the Maryland Legislature and signed into law by Governor Millard Tawes. I became the only dentist in the United States who could practice medical (and dental) anesthesiology by special act of the legislature.

Instead of going back into the hospital practice of anesthesiology I decided to remain in dentistry. I utilized my anesthesia talents and initiated the idea of placing patients under the influence of intravenous drugs to alleviate fear and anxiety and repaired all of their teeth in one sitting while the patient relaxed in a euphoric state known as conscious sedation. The word of this service spread rapidly throughout Maryland. After 16 years of practice I was able to retire. I sold my practice but within weeks I was coaxed out of retirement by an offer to teach those concepts of conscious sedation, which I pioneered, to dentists and medical residents in anesthesiology at the Johns Hopkins Hospital. The year was 1979.

My first day in the operating rooms at Johns Hopkins was like no other experience in operating rooms I had ever been in. During the two decades of my anesthesia years I had worked in the operating room of almost every hospital in Baltimore, except Hopkins. What was the big difference?

The difference was not in the physical surroundings. It was a state of mind, an excitement, the realization of a childhood dream come true. This dream had its origins at age 14 while a high school student at the Baltimore City College.

I used to gaze out of the window of my history classroom in City's second floor from which I could see the enormous Johns Hopkins Medical Institution off in the distance. I dreamed of one day working there, and fantasized about a future in medicine at that institution. These fantasies were so compelling that one day during my senior year at City, I went by streetcar to the Hopkins Hospital. I took the elevator to the eighth floor of the Blalock Building on which were the observation entrances to the operating rooms on the seventh floor. In these small, dressing rooms were gowns, caps and masks for visiting physicians. Without making inquiries as to the permissibility of what I was about to do, I donned a gown, mask and cap and walked into the first operating room I came to. My gown and mask disguise shielded my age. I sat on a long bench located almost four feet above the operating floor, fenced in by a railing and hiding behind my mask, I watched my first operation. The surgeon was Dr. Walter Dandy, a Hopkins pioneer in brain surgery, and the sight I saw almost overwhelmed me. I was so impressed that I wrote an essay on my experiences which I handed in as an English class assignment at City College. It read as follows:

CRANIOTOMY FOR A BRAIN TUMOR

"Her head completely shaved, a rather well built, middle aged woman, was wheeled into the operating room of the Johns Hopkins Hospital. Nurses were busily engaged in preparing the room for the entrance of the famous brain surgeon, Dr. Walter Dandy. Iodine in great quantities was liberally spread over the entire scalp, as the anesthetist proceeded to etherize the patient with a mask, using a can of Squibb's ether, drop by drop on the cotton mask. Complicated equipment lined the walls of the room, making the room resemble a broadcasting station, with tiny blue lights, and red lights, and dials, and tubes for the operation of the electric knife, the electric cauterizer, and the bone drill.

Suddenly Dr. Dandy walked into the room. An average-sized man, wearing bone-rimmed glasses, quite ordinary in appearance. He simply wore a shirt, and white pants, no rubber gloves, or mask and gown. A scalpel was immediately handed to him. He palpated the patient's head, then made four superficial incisions into the shaved scalp where he expected to cut away the bone . . . He then threw the knife onto a table and walked out of the operating room. His assistants quickly began to prepare the patient for the main part of the operation by swabbing up the blood oozing out of the superficial incision which Dr. Dandy had just made. The patient finally was completely covered with sterile sheets, clamped to each other, her head lying to one side, the right side up. The nurse anesthetist was also completely covered as if in a tent, while she continued to administer the ether. The lights in the room were turned off, the shades drawn down over the huge bay windows, and a spotlight lit up the surgical site.

Dr. Dandy, completely masked, gowned, with snugly fitting rubber gloves, entered the room, nodded greetings to the visitors in the small gallery, and sat on a white metal stool in front of the patient's head. Every part of the patient and anesthetist was completely covered with sterile sheets, except the small area where Dr. Dandy had made his location incisions. He was handed a scalpel. Very quickly he dissected away the skin covering the section of bone which he expected to open. Numerous arteries began to bleed profusely, but these were rapidly clamped by two assistants. The flesh was now drawn back into a flap. The boney skull was exposed directly above the ear and temple, covering an area of about three square inches, or about the area covered by the bottom of a milk bottle. There, glistening in the light emitted from the single powerful electric bulb which Dr. Dandy wore attached by a head band to his head, was the dull, moist, whitish yellow bone of the skull. The area was now clean, completely free of blood, it was now time to begin drilling the holes in the skull so that access could be made to the brain.

An assistant handed an electric drill to the surgeon. In it was a bit about $1/2$ inch in diameter. The motor was turned on, and Dr. Dandy explained that he never uses an electric drill, but some company wanted him to try it to see if it was superior to the hand drill. The whirling drill was placed next to the bone very carefully, but as in drilling a piece of metal, the bit began to slide over the bone, and would not remain steady. In addition, the drill suddenly locked, and would not rotate, due probably to the fact that all the oil was eliminated previously during the time it was sterilized. Dr. Dandy dispensed with this, and used his hand drill, which is nothing more than a brace and bit which he turned by hand. As he applied pressure to the brace while turning it, tiny bone shavings which resembled saw dust spread about and occupied the region about the bit. He drilled four of these holes, each about $1/2$inch in diameter, and when he approached the covering of the brain, known as the dura mater, he proceeded with the utmost delicacy. He next used an instrument, resembling a curved awl, and proceeded to carefully cut through the final tiny layer of bone which separated the brain covering from the air. He did this in each hole separately. Then he pushed the awl from one hole, till it appeared at the opposite one. A flexible saw blade, in wire form about the size of a piece of string in diameter, was attached to a minute hook in the end of the awl. The saw blade was then drawn back thru the two holes. Dr. Dandy then grasped the two ends of the blade, and with a steady back and forth motion, sawed thru the bone. The blades broke several times, causing the surgeon to curse, the "damned American process of metal manufacture", since he could no longer order his superior foreign brand. (Hitler was in charge of Nazi Germany at that time.)

In a few moments the bone was completely sawed away, leaving one end attached to the flesh covering the scalp. This was turned back, out of the way, and covered with gauze soaked in some saline solution. The brain was not visible yet. It was encased in a grayish, fibrous, tough covering known as the dura mater, however it seemed to bulge out of the opening in the skull.

Then with a tiny, sharp scalpel, and with a feathery touch, Dr. Dandy, made a minute incision into the dura mater. There was not a sound in the operating room. One could hear a pin drop. Very gently he proceeded to cut away the covering around the exposed area of the brain, and this too, was folded back against the piece of bone as a flap. There, the brain was now exposed. A feeling of admiration for this surgeon came over me. A helpless, sort of depression also enveloped me momentarily as I gazed at the brain, pulsating with each heart beat as if it were going to bulge out of the skull any second. It was glistening, pinkish yellow-gray, with thousands of blood vessels running all over it. I paused and thought how tremendous, and marvelous and mysterious this was, this great controlling mechanism of our varied complex emotions, and feelings, and actions. There it was, exposed in the living state, bulging, and pulsating with life.

The purpose of the operation was to remove a tumor which was growing around the optic nerve, in the region of the pituitary gland or hypophysis. This growth had caused the patient to become totally blind, due to excessive pressure on the nerve. Now the nerve and the pituitary gland is located at the base of the brain, at a point about two inches in back of the forehead, on a level with the top of the ear lobe, approximately. In order to reach this region, Dr. Dandy simply inserted a curved piece of blunt, shiny metal, one-half inch wide and about three inches long. With this, he gently separated the brain from its covering, wherever bleeding occurred he cauterized it, and with a minimum of pressure he pushed the brain aside so as to expose the tumor, the optic nerve, and the pituitary gland. The tumor was nothing more than a grayish yellow growth, rather vascular, which resembled brain tissue. It was in such proximity to the optic nerve that Dr. Dandy had to, with a tiny blade, cut the optic nerve leading to the right eye. This nerve is the largest of the cranial nerves, being about $1/4$ inch in diameter. He cut it by running the small knife across it. The knife seemed to melt through it. Then with small forceps, he proceeded to remove the tumor piece-meal from the nerve. It took Dr. Dandy about 15 minutes to remove all of the tumor which was the size of a small hazel nut. When it was completely removed, a mild saline solution was squirted into the cavity around the brain, it was drained out, the dura mater was closed and the bone was replaced. The operation was over. It took two hours to perform. The patient will now be able to see out of one eye."

It has been 45 years since I had been in the Hopkins operating rooms, and here I was, fulfilling an unrequited dream of childhood, not as a medical student, not as an intern, not as a resident, but as a professor in full regalia of green scrub suit, mask, cap and a white coat. On that first day I floated through that (now ultramodern) long tiled hallway of 15 operating rooms on the 7th floor of Blalock and somehow I could not escape the fantasy that I was still that 14 year old City College student. I really did not belong here. Was I still hiding behind my cap and mask?

Despite the fact that I had been working in operating rooms in Baltimore Hospitals for over 18 years; that I was more at home in operating rooms than my own home, somehow the realization of a dream come true did not materialize. I was still simply 14 again. I could not wipe away the smile behind my mask.

It wasn't until some of the surgeons with whom I had worked in other hospitals greeted me that reality finally set in.

There's something so satisfying about the final realization of an old dream. And on this first day I lived and fondled each moment of it. It was possible to do this since I was not distracted by the anesthesia necessities of the moment. I was simply "casing the joint" familiarizing myself with the equipment in preparation for my forthcoming teaching duties which were scheduled to start the next day.

Prior to 1980, anesthesiology at Johns Hopkins was primarily directed by nurse anesthetists. With the appointment of Donald R. Benson, Eugene Nagel, and then Mark Rogers as Chairman of the department, the specialty underwent a radical metamorphosis.

For the first time in its history, research in anesthesiology instead of simply clinical instruction, was emphasized. Within a few years the department became the largest anesthesiology training center in the world with over 50 physician residents in training and over 40 professors training the residents. The department name was changed to reflect two specialties. It became The Department of Anesthesiology and Critical Care Medicine. There were so many operating rooms that it was necessary to retain the nurse anesthetists to aid in the operation of this gigantic undertaking. My job was to train both the oral surgical and physician anesthesia residents in the entire concept of conscious sedation.

Conscious sedation involved an approach to managing patients undergoing surgery who would be conscious during the operation but would not remember the event. It involved behavioral conditioning, a fancy phrase for developing an intimate personal rapport with the patient. The concept was based in part on the Chinese approach to electrical acupuncture wherein the patient was mentally conditioned for two days before the operation and instructed in how he should conduct himself in the operating room. In China he was instructed not to talk, move his body, kick his legs, or even scratch his nose if it itched and no matter what he felt he was not to complain. Chinese patients were selected specifically for acupuncture after they passed a simple test which revealed whether or not they were hypnotizable or suggestible. For example: they were asked to clasp their hands together while their eyes were closed. Imaginary glue was

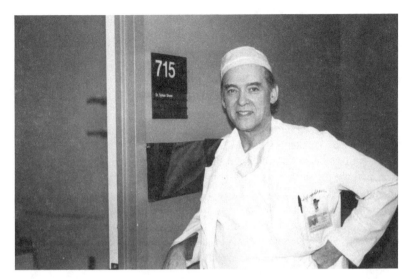

Outside my office at the Johns Hopkins Hospital.

placed between their fingers. They were told by the acupuncturist that the glue was setting and that it would be impossible to unclasp their hands. They were then told to "try" to unclasp their hands. If they could not free one hand from the other, the patient was considered sufficiently suggestible to undergo surgery under acupuncture. For the next two days an intimate relationship between the acupuncturist and the patient was developed. The patient was told he would be looked after, cared for, that he would not have to go to sleep, therefore, he would not have to wake up which was much safer than going to sleep. He would be awake throughout the operation, but he would not mind any type of discomfort. No drugs were to be used, and the only thing he would feel would be two or three small needle sticks in his hand between his thumb and first finger, and another in his ear, or toe or arm.

Through the needles would run a mild electric current which was supposed to help alleviate any pain.

I spent a month in China in 1975 studying acupuncture for surgical anesthesia and discovered that only 30 per cent of surgery is done under acupuncture. Seventy per cent was performed under "western" type anesthesia, meaning inhaled gases for total unconsciousness under general or under spinal anesthesia. Why only 30 per cent? Why not 40 or 50 per cent? But the 30 per cent figure was firm.

Upon my return to the United States I discussed this with Dr. Jacob Conn, a Professor of Psychiatry at Hopkins who was the foremost hypnotherapist in Maryland. Upon learning of this 30 per-cent figure in China he said, "Sylvan, do you know only 30 out of 100 patients are hypnotizable. The other 70 per cent will not go under."

I also learned that it makes no difference where the acupuncture needles are inserted. The purpose of the needles with the flow of a mild electric current serves only one purpose—to cause the elaboration of morphine-like substances known as endorphines. These substances might assist suggestion in that the endorphines cause the pain threshold to rise, thus making the pain of surgery somewhat more tolerable.

With conscious sedation we use a similar type of intensive suggestion but no electric needles. We do, however, use intravenous drugs to obliterate memory but not consciousness. To obliterate pain we employ local anesthesia with Xylocaine, but the patient cannot remember the pain of the needles injecting the local anesthetic. This method is effective in almost 100 per cent of patients.

After telling the patients that they are not to talk, move or scratch their noses, we tell them why. The "why" is the motivating explanation to be certain they follow our instructions. We tell them that if they talk or move, or kick their legs or even wiggle their toes, their blood pressure may go up and this will result in excessive bleeding. We show them a clipping from the Baltimore Sun newspaper which reads:

TALKING RAISES
BLOOD PRESSURE
AT LEAST 10%

The reading of this clipping reinforces what we have just told the patient.

In the operating room we inject three drugs intravenously. A narcotic such as Demerol, a tranquilizer such as Atarax, and Brevital.

These drugs are given in a very minute, measured dose, which obliterates memory but not consciousness for about 8 to 10 minutes during which time the surgeon injects the local anesthetic in the site to be operated. Amnesia can be detected by divergence of the eyeballs. Following the 8- to 10-minute period of amnesia, the patient enters a 1 1/2 hour period of pleasant euphoria without the necessity for any additional intravenous drugs. The local anesthetic obliterates the pain of surgery. The intravenous drugs also eliminate every vestige of apprehension, anxiety and nervousness. The preoperative verbal behavioral indoctrination about

THE SUN, Monday, June 8, 1981

Talking raises blood pressure at least 10%,

By Mary Knudson

A University of Maryland research group has found that talking makes a person's blood pressure rise significantly, a factor not now taken into account in blood pressure testing.

If blood pressures were taken while patients talked, more people would be told they are hypertensive, says Dr. James J. Lynch, professor and director of the psychophysiological clinic at University Hospital.

The finding also is important for the 23 million Americans whose high blood pressure already is diagnosed, Dr. Lynch said in an interview. "The higher the baseline pressure, the more the pressure goes up when you speak," he said.

The rise in blood pressure occurred when people talked, when babies cried, when deaf people communicated in sign language, when children read aloud in classrooms and even when people were asked to read aloud in a room by themselves. The average rise was between 10 percent and 20 percent, an increase Dr. Lynch termed "significant."

Clipping from the BALTIMORE SUN of June 8, 1981 which we permit the patient to read to emphasize why they should not talk during surgery under conscious sedation, since a rise in blood pressure could induce bleeding.

the necessity for complete relaxation to diminish bleeding then takes over and the patient remains unmoving, not speaking, cooperative and relaxed for the duration of the operation.

This is what I was supposed to be teaching. This is not what always happened.

The residents in oral surgery were eager learners. The third-and fourth-year medical students were hungry for knowledge and were apt pupils at my lectures.

But the physician residents in anesthesia were totally indifferent to this aspect of anesthesia practice. There were several reasons for this apathy.

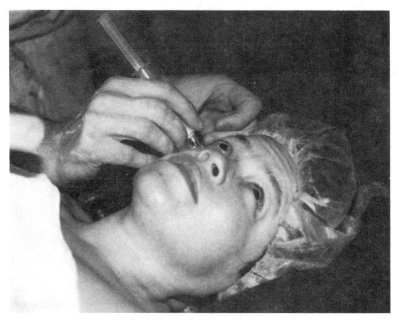

This patient who is to undergo cataract surgery for the right eye is receiving a retro-bulbar local block. Divergence of her eyeballs indicates that memory is temporarily abolished under conscious sedation anesthesia.

First, conscious sedation was not a requirement for residency training. General anesthesia, spinal, epidural, endotracheal, were all required by American Anesthesia Specialty Boards and each case was recorded on the computers to the credit of the resident. Each resident had to administer a certain number of spinals, generals, etc. But there was no space on the computer for conscious sedation.

Secondly, conscious sedation required time, communication and the development of rapport between doctor and patient. In the operating room the success or failure of the ability to develop rapport and empathy with the patient was immediately evident. If the patient was quiet and cooperative it was successful. If the patient became irritable, restless, and unduly apprehensive, the resident failed. The fear of failure was prevalent when a resident attempted conscious sedation but not with general anesthesia. With general the patient was immediately unconscious after a large intravenous shot of Pentothal. No talking was necessary, no empathy, no rapport, there was apparent success every time.

The word "apparent" is used since success was not always present

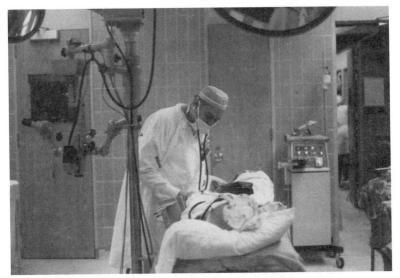

Administering conscious sedation anesthesia at the Johns Hopkins Hospital.

after a large dose of Pentothal was injected into a patient. There were complications such as spasm of the vocal chords known as laryngeal spasm, vomiting, fall in blood pressure, an erratic pulse. The patient, however, was unconscious and knew nothing about these induction complications. In most instances the resident could cover up the complication from the eyes of the surgeon who was still scrubbing. But the resident did not have to talk to the patient and waste his good time.

This is what I was faced with when I began to teach conscious sedation at Hopkins.

The fact that the patient was awake and did not have to wake up, that he was far safer from a life and death standpoint was not a priority with the resident. He wanted only to fulfill his requirements and conscious sedation was not one of them.

The oral surgery residents were eager to learn all aspects of this method since this is what they would employ in their dental practice. They didn't want patients to be sleepy after an anesthetic since their patients were all outpatients who had to get up and leave the dental office.

The physician resident didn't care. His general anesthesia patients were carted off to a recovery room and kept over night or several days depending on the severity of the operation.

I would enter an operating room where the patient was to undergo a hernioplasty or a D & C or a hemorrhoidectomy. After getting the surgeon's ok for conscious sedation, I would indicate to the resident or nurse anesthetist that I would like to join them to do this patient under conscious sedation. Immediately a confrontation would ensue, and the tension of opposition to my request was so thick it could be cut with a knife. I brought this to the attention of the Director of all anesthesia services. He immediately issued a memorandum to all the professors, residents, students, and nurse anesthetists. The letter follows:

THE JOHNS HOPKINS UNIVERSITY

SCHOOL OF MEDICINE

Robert T. Donham, M.D.
Director, Anesthesia Services
Department of Anesthesiology/Critical Care Medicine

July 17, 1981

Please address reply care of
THE JOHNS HOPKINS HOSPITAL
BALTIMORE, MARYLAND 21205
(301) 955-8465

MEMORANDUM TO: Attending Anesthesiologists
                      Residents
                      CRNA's
                      SRNA's

FROM: Robert T. Donham, M.D.
                      Director
                      Anesthesia Services

SUBJECT: Conscious Sedation Techniques By Dr. Sylvan Shane

        Dr. Sylvan Shane is conducting a research project involving conscious sedation and behavioral technology on patients posted as local standby. This project is aimed at furthering the total capabilities of the various members of our Staff. At present it is indeed in a research stage and has been properly discussed and approved by appropriate members of the Senior Staff. Dr. Shane is uniquely qualified to conduct such a study and it is hoped that the results will add significantly to the armamentarium of techniques of this Department.

        I am requesting that Dr. Shane be given full cooperation whenever and wherever he indicates he wishes to take over a local standby anesthetic whether it be in the GOR, Gyn, Wilmer, FCC, or Oral Surgery. He would be delighted to have any member of our Staff observe and/or assist him during the procedures. However, Dr. Shane will assume full responsibility for these cases.

        I would encourage you to whenever possible, avail yourselves of the opportunity to observe and/or participate in the techniques Dr. Shane is researching. At present, the results seem to be very promising. As with any anesthetic technique and/or medical advancement, a period of appropriately controlled and monitored clinical research is necessary to establish the efficacy. The techniques which Dr. Shane is utilizing deserve to be appropriately and completely tested.

RTD:jt

Memorandum sent to the anesthesia staff at the Johns Hopkins Hospital regarding my research project involving conscious sedation.

This memorandum worked like magic. When I entered an operating room it was as if the president of the university had walked in. That is what I wanted, however, another problem arose. The resident or nurse anesthetist simply walked out of the room and left me there to do the case myself. After several weeks of this it appeared as if a conspiracy were in progress. I was there to teach conscious sedation to students, not to administer it myself.

When I realized that the medical residents were simply not interested, I discussed the problem with the professor in charge. The old adage about leading a horse to water was dragged out. "One day the anesthesia boards will make this a requirement," he said, "in the meantime there isn't much we can do." He pointed out that there was another problem that was subtle in nature and difficult to document. This was the fact that I was a D.D.S. and not an M.D. and that the M.D. residents already had an ego-shattering problem with having the nurse anesthetists doing the same work as the residents did and in most instances doing it more efficiently because of their years of experience. Many of these residents were already specialists in pediatrics, internal medicine and cardiology. Many had already been out in practice, with an office and secretaries, and having given all that up to train in anesthesiology, they were then faced with being trained by a D.D.S. This may be too ego-shattering for some of them. We know it exists when a nurse anesthetist is instructed to supervise them. The professor indicated he wished he had an answer to this unique but subtle problem that exists in no other specialty of medicine except anesthesiology.

I decided that if the residents wanted to learn the fine details of conscious sedation they would have to seek me out. In the meantime I decided to begin to evaluate the possibilities of conscious sedation in more complex operations which had never before been explored in detail.

For two years I worked to perfect the use of conscious sedation in D & C's, the laparoscopy operation and in opthalmologic surgery.

The laparaoscopy procedure was the most difficult of all operations to perform under conscious sedation. Why was this so?

Laparoscopy means examination of the interior of the abdominal cavity by means of a laparoscope. The laparoscope is a long hollow tube, one-half inch in diameter, with an electric bulb at one end, a microscopic eyepiece at the other end. The laparoscopy examination is performed by pushing the sharp end of the laparoscope through the area of the umbilicus and into the abdominal cavity without having to cut the patient open to make a diagnosis. It is also used to sterilize the female by pulling a trigger attached to the side of the instrument which snaps a plastic ring around the fallopian tube, thus rendering her sterile.

When this tube is inserted into the abdomen it is difficult to distinguish individual organs since everything is so bunched together. It is, therefore, necessary to get the intestines out of the way. Two things are done to accomplish this. The operating table is slanted so that the patient's head is towards the floor and her legs up toward the ceiling. This position known as Trendelenburg, permits the intestines to bunch up under the diaphragm, leaving the pelvic organs such as the uterus, fallopian tubes and bladder exposed to view through the laparoscope. To enhance the view, carbon dioxide gas is blown into the cavity by attaching a rubber tube from a tank of carbon dioxide to a nipple on the side arm of the laparoscope. The abdomen is then blown up like a balloon. Carbon dioxide which will not explode, is used instead of oxygen in the event of an electrical spark which could ignite oxygen and explode.

Two things occur when the patient is distended by carbon dioxide gas: the intestines are impacted up against her diaphragm; the diaphragm is pressed up against the lower border of the heart, which may limit the force of its beat. The patient's breathing is impaired because of the upward pressure. In addition, the carbon dioxide is being absorbed into her blood stream which lowers the ph of her blood, making it acid in reaction instead of neutral. When blood is rendered acid it sets the stage for cardiac arrest. These disadvantages are all enhanced by rendering the patient unconscious under general anesthesia, wherein the patient loses all control of the protective reflexes.

I found that by performing this operation under conscious sedation the patient could not only go home the same day, but the dangers from carbon dioxide absorption and the strained upside down position did not affect the patient in the deleterious manner caused by general anesthesia. Under conscious sedation the patient was awake and did not have to wake up. The imminence of death was remote since her protective reflexes were operating and not depressed by the general anesthetic.

When the laparoscopy operation was performed under general anesthesia in third world or developing countries, the spectre of death hovered over every laparoscopy operation. Deaths were so numerous that an organization at Hopkins known as JHPIEGO* contacted me to request that I travel to various third world countries to teach this conscious sedation method to anesthesiologists and anesthesia technicians. All expenses would be paid and in addition I would receive a stipend for each trip.

---

*JHPIEGO means the Johns Hopkins Program for International Education in Gynecology and Obstetrics.

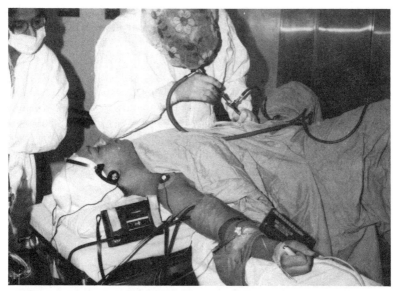

Patient undergoing laparoscopy under conscious sedation at the Johns Hopkins Hospital. In her hand is a switch which if compressed causes the BEEPOPHONE (the black box next to her hand) to beep, telling the surgeon she is uncomfortable. On her ears are earphones through which she listens to music from the tape recorder at her right shoulder.

JHPIEGO was financed by the United States Government Foreign Aid Mission and the objective was to aid in reducing the size of families in Africa, the Near East, and South America, as a way of reducing starvation in these countries. JHPIEGO was sending gynecologists to these countries to instruct in the use of the laparoscope for sterilization. They even supplied the laparoscopes which cost thousands of dollars. When a death from anesthesia occurred the news spread rapidly through the village, and the natives would no longer patronize the program.

JHPIEGO officials knew that the possibility of death was remote with the conscious sedation method. As a result I was requested to travel to such places as Tunisia, Morocco, and The Cameroons, to teach Moslems and blacks the fine points of conscious sedation.

My experiences in Tunisia are recorded in a prior book entitled FROM POLE TO POLE AND BETWEEN. This was published in 1984. In Chapter Five there is a description of my experiences in 1984 in the Cameroons, a nation on the West Coast of Africa, near the Equator and not far from the Congo.

Anesthesia practice has changed radically since the use of nitrous oxide or laughing gas in 1844 by a dentist, Horace Wells, and the discovery of ether as an anesthetic by another dentist, William T. G. Morton in 1846. From 1846 until 1943 ether was the king of anesthetics even though numerous anesthetics were discovered in the intervening years. Anesthetics such as chloroform, Pentothal, ethylene, cyclopropane, Metopryl and the halogenated anesthetics such as halothane were introduced but none could topple ether's superior position. The reason for this was the ability of ether to relax abdominal muscles sufficiently to prevent the intestines from bulging out during abdominal surgery, a condition which the surgeon could not tolerate. Ether was the only drug capable of producing this intense degree of muscle relaxation safely. Yet ether's side effects made it the most undesirable of anesthetics. Ether caused postoperative nausea and vomiting, sometimes for days; prolonged recovery and predisposed patients to pneumonia and atelectasis. Ether remained king not from choice but from the necessity to provide abdominal relaxation.

In 1943, ether lost its kingly crown, being toppled by a drug known as curare. Curare was not an anesthetic. It was a muscle relaxant which when injected intravenously in combination with a more innocuous anesthetic such as Pentothal, or cyclopropane, or halothane could produce abdominal relaxation without the sickening, side effects of ether.

The year 1943 was the year of the anesthesia revolution. By 1987 inflammable anesthetics such as ether and cyclopropane were banned from almost every hospital in the United States by insurance companies who refused to insure institutions who used explosive anesthetics.

The administration of anesthetics is only as safe as the administrator. The expert in this specialty is the individual who can crawl inside the anesthetized patient's cardiovascular system and intuitively know what's going on. This intuitive grasp is not learned from books or medical journals. It becomes an integral part of the anesthesiologist's inner being only after many years of clinical experience. There are some anesthesiologists who never develop this intuitive understanding. These are the individuals who are never certain from minute to minute as to the physiological homeostatic status of the patient. They are nervous, insecure, fearful, and never seem to overcome the fear of losing a patient. I could identify these individuals since they seemed to be in perpetual motion during an operation checking and rechecking the patient's pulse, blood pressure and respiration, color of their fingernails, etc.

I distinctly remember my own feelings of insecurity when I was appointed chief of the department of anesthesiology at the South Baltimore

General Hospital upon completion of my anesthesia residency in Camden, New Jersey. During my residency my chief was the one who was ultimately responsible for my errors. In anesthesia practice an error can be fatal. I completed my residency on June 30, 1945 and on July 1st I was suddenly on my own in Baltimore, with no chief to back me up or take responsibility if a patient should die on the operating table, or simply never regain consciousness after an anesthetic. My job was to escort the patients down the long, dark corridor of unconsciousness and then return them back to light and consciousness. One unexplained failure in this endeavor and my career in anesthesia could end—just like that. In hospitals, there is usually no second chance when death occurs for which there is no logical explanation. I was especially vulnerable since my degree was in dentistry and not in medicine. It took four years of clinical practice before I was totally at ease in the operating room. I remember this, even to the exact date. It happened suddenly. One morning I turned the key to my ignition en route to the hospital, and suddenly the anxiety and apprehension that I was experiencing each day was no longer there. It was as if a curtain had lifted and I just knew within me that no matter how sick the patient, nor how serious the surgery, I could manage it with total confidence. A weight was suddenly lifted and I actually felt ebullient.

During my early years in anesthesia, monitors were unknown. Today the patient's heart and pulse are monitored by an EKG machine which displays the heart beat on a TV monitor screen. The pulse can be heard as a rhythmic beep, beep, and the oxygen concentration in the blood can be monitored by means of a tiny infra-red, bearing clip which fits on the finger. Blood pressure is taken automatically and recorded on a tape like an adding machine. Residents training in anesthesia in 1987 are being monitor-trained, meaning that if the monitor breaks down or malfunctions they are frequently at a loss to determine intuitively at what point the patient is in her unconscious journey. With mechanical monitors the anesthesia trainee seldom has to touch the patient, and I do believe that the intuitive aspect of his training tends to suffer. Monitors are frequently highly essential as illustrated by the following case at the Johns Hopkins Hospital involving a three-year-old little boy with a brain tumor. Treatment required X-ray radiation to his brain every day for 30 days. For the first five days he was rendered totally unconscious with Halothane, an inhalational anesthetic, then paralyzed with curare to facilitate the insertion of an endotracheal tube into his windpipe. After five days of this trauma to the child's vocal cords, and the parent's complaint of his post operative nausea, vomiting and sleeplessness because of the Halothane, I

ANESTHESIA PROGRESS

A Journal for Pain and Anxiety Control

CASE REPORT:

CONSCIOUS SEDATION ADMINISTERED DAILY FOR 25 DAYS IN A 3 YEAR OLD CHILD

Sylvan M. Shane, D.D.S.

Department of Anesthesiology and Critical Care Medicine, The John Hopkins University School of Medicine, Baltimore Maryland

A three year old male child with a brain tumor in the right frontal lobe required daily radiation therapy for 30 days in a attempt to shrink the tumor. The child was a major management problem who cried and resisted hospital personnel. The patient had received steroid therapy for a year which produced an edematous condition which obscured all veins in the arms, legs and neck. Each radiation session lasted 40 minutes to an hour during which time the child had to lie face down in a custom built, lead lined plaster cradle which held his head in a secure position so that the x-ray beam struck only the tumor. Any slight movement would have caused the beam to strike the optic nerve which would have resulted in blindness. It was of paramount importance that the child not move during the hour radiation session.

tal methohexital plus intramuscular ketamine was employed but this resulted in uncontrolled movement after 15 minutes since the child had an enormously high tolerance for both barbiturates and ketamine.

The technique which solved the problem was one that had been previously employed by the author in managing mentally retarded children requiring extensive restorative dental procedures. The child was given a sub-anesthetic dose of ketamine, 2½ mg per pound, mixed with hydroxyzine hydrochloride (Vistaril) 25 mg, plus .01 mg of glycopyrrolate (Robinul). These drugs were mixed in one syringe and injected in the buttock. Hydroxyzine was employed to potentiate both the ketamine and the glycopyrrolate, to reduce the tendency to vomit, and to act

Title of the published paper describing the administration of conscious sedation in a three-year-old for 25 days in succession.

was called into this case to determine if conscious sedation could be used instead of general anesthesia. One of the main concerns was use of the endotracheal tube for the next 25 days, since this could cause permanent injury to his vocal cords.

Although the radiation session involved no pain, it was essential that the child remain absolutely motionless while lying face down on his abdomen, for a period of 45 minutes. The slightest movement of his head could deflect the radiation beam from the tumor to his optic nerve which could result in blindness. In addition, neither I nor anyone else, could be in the lead-lined radiation chamber so that we would not be radiated ourselves. I had to observe the child through a remote television hook-up and watch for any untoward reaction on a Sony TV monitor screen. I could see and hear his heart beat on a remote EKG monitor. The radiation technician could in a second shut off the X-ray beam if I had to rush back into the lead-lined room.

I placed the child under intravenous conscious sedation, and attached a small rubber anesthesia mask over his nose and mouth through which he breathed a dilute mixture of laughing gas, not enough to produce unconsciousness—but enough to produce mental repose.

I had employed and taught this method while teaching at the Medical University of South Carolina on mentally incompetent children requiring extensive dental repair. For the next 25 days the child underwent his daily radiation therapy. The child was wide awake within two minutes of discontinuing the laughing gas. There were no after effects, no nausea, no vomiting, no nightmares, and no vocal cord damage since no endotracheal tube was used. And above all, there was no movement of the child's head or body during the radiation.

After 14 days of this daily routine, I decided to make a motion picture film of this event since it was so reliably predictable. This case was reported in an anesthesia journal in 1984.*

The hiatus of my career in anesthesia occurred in Chicago when I was selected as the recipient for the 1985 Heidbrink Award. This award is given annually by the American Dental Society of Anesthesiology to the physician or dentist who has made the greatest contribution to the specialty of anesthesiology. In my acceptance speech I roamed over much of the critical material already described in this chapter. I stressed that if dentists were to be trained in conscious sedation in the future, the dental schools themselves would have to assume the responsibility. We could no longer depend upon the physician anesthesiologist, with his plethora of egotistical hang-ups to train dentists of the future in managing the fear and anxiety-stricken dental patient with conscious sedation.

---

*Shane, Sylvan: Conscious Sedation, Administered Daily for 25 Days in a 3-Year-Old Child. Anesthesia Progress. Mar-Apr. Page 85–86 1984.

CHAPTER III

THE CAMEROONS AND PARIS

In July 1984, the JHPIEGO organization at Johns Hopkins sent me to The Cameroons in Africa to instruct their medical personnel in the fine points of conscious sedation as applied to the laparoscopy operation, a procedure used mainly to sterilize females and thereby control the enormous population explosion in that country.

Since these were my retirement years I decided to cross the Atlantic by ship instead of by air en route to the Cameroons.

Crossing the Atlantic in a luxury vessel is a true five-day vacation. As I sit alone on the upper deck of the Cunard's Queen Elizabeth, far from the security of land, in the middle of the Atlantic's grandeur, I sense the earth's rotundity, the frailness of human life and the presence of the chilling winds. Unlike earthbound man, the imminence of danger lies everpresent in the quiet of the conscious mind, just beyond the ships railings, and constantly reinforced by life boats suspended from their davits. Perhaps this element of danger lends to the excitement of going out to sea. But there's something more—there's the serenity, the peace, the sense of motion, the ultimate destination, the great dome of blue overhead, the intimate contact with the Eternal that is difficult to achieve on the Baltimore Beltway.

I sit on a rear deck and am fascinated by the light blue wake, churned up by the ship's twin propellers. I read for a page or two then look out to the horizon surrounding me, where the sky dips down into the sea. I cannot "look the other way and see two Islands in a bay" as did Edna St. Vincent Milay in her poem *Renaissance*. Here it's only the deep, dark, blue sea, nothing else. It is far beyond the range of the sea gull, and devoid of the Antarctic gales which support the earth-circling flights of the magnificent Albatross. No life is here except for that unseen predatory population which exists beneath the surface of the watery deep. And the sunsets at sea are indescribably magnificent.

The ship's route is a northeasterly direction towards Newfoundland after which it heads out directly east to England. The northeasterly direction is shorter since it takes advantage of the narrower circumferance of

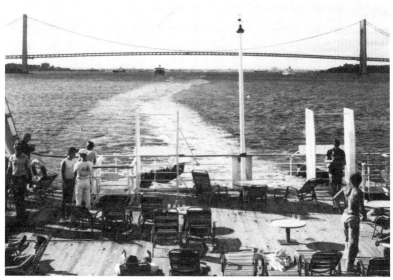

From the rear deck of the Queen Elizabeth II, the Verrezano Bridge and the towers of New York disappear in the distance as I head for England.

the earth which exists the closer we approach the North Pole. The fact that we are heading north mocks the month of July and midsummer. The North Atlantic is always cold. Even in the bright sunlight, sweaters and blankets are essential.

Meals are sumptuous and gourmet, sleep is profound and easy, and the days pass too quickly in rapid succession. There are two films each day at 4 and 9 P.M. in a theatre larger than most theatres in Baltimore, and a library which puts the smaller branches of the Enoch Pratt to shame. There are five dining rooms, and in the largest, a special section for Kosher dining, with dairy dishes for breakfast and lunch and meat dishes for supper. Activities include lectures, several supervised exercise areas, steam rooms and saunas with expert masseurs, a Las Vegas gambling area not unlike the Sands in Vegas. This area opens when the ship is beyond the 50 mile limit from New York. There is a multitude of shops all with I. Magnin quality and prices, and a fully-equipped hospital with operating rooms. The ship is longer than three football fields. It is 13 stories high and travels through the Atlantic at 30 miles an hour, with far less motion than an Amtrak passenger train. I did not mention the discos, multiple orchestras, night clubs, beauty salons, swimming pools, both indoor and outdoor, six elevators, and bars too numerous to mention. The alcoholic would be in seventh heaven on this ship.

There are over 2,000 passengers on board which creates quite a headache for British passport control once the ship reaches England. To circumvent this they fly a customs official to New York, he boards the ship, and handles all the passport stamping and formalities before the ship reaches England. On Monday he sees all passengers from decks 1 and 2. On Tuesday passengers from 3 and 4, etc.

To give some idea of how the QE-2 feeds its passengers, the chief steward revealed to me what he purchases for each crossing.

Milk	22,000 pounds
Eggs	80,000
Fresh Fruit	22,000 pounds
Cream	3,000 quarts
Butter	3,500 pounds
Sugar	5,000 pounds
Flour	3,000 pounds
Wine and Beer	16,000 bottles
Cheeses	3,000 pounds
Chicken	5,000
Cigarettes	25,000 packages

After four days at sea I was still referring to the ship's direction map to show me how to get from here to there. The ship is like a gigantic maze.

I sit in the magnificent theatre, complete with balcony, waiting for the film "Terms of Endearment" to start. I am five minutes too early. I suddenly become aware of the life of the ship—a slight motion, first to the right then seconds later to the left. Then I become aware of an intermittent vibration through the theatre seat, reminiscent of the beginnings of an earthquake which I once experienced in Los Angeles. The theatre curtains sway ever so slightly as the ship rolls from port to starboard.

Most of the passengers are older, over 60, since younger people cannot afford $2,000 for a one-way trip across the Atlantic. Flying across in five hours instead of five days costs as little as $189.00. As a result, airborne passenger traffic will eventually antiquate the luxury ocean liner.

The peaceful invigorating experience of sunsets at sea, of just sitting on deck and experiencing the vast, dark blue Atlantic, the beautiful sunrises, and finally as we approached the coast of England there appeared the first

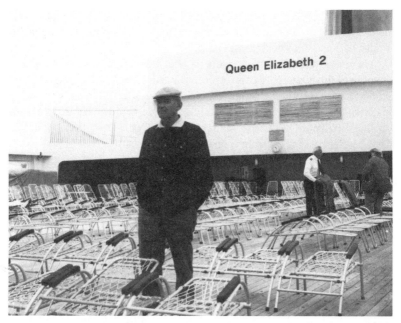

Relaxing on the upper deck of the Queen Elizabeth 2 as I head for England across the Atlantic.

lone seagull, long before land was sighted, and I knew that the good earth was just beyond the horizon.

England seemed to poke its head up out of the sea. At first it was a speck that grew larger the closer the ship approached. Then, in time, it began to take shape. A long finger of land with a lighthouse appeared and, as we climbed over the horizon, it grew broader and broader, then greener and greener, then there were more seagulls, and sailing ships, and tiny houses, then farms, and freighters and docks and we were there.

I spent the first day walking London. I followed the Strand which parallels the Thames River. I crossed Westminster Bridge and gazed at Big Ben and the houses of Parliament. I returned by way of St. Paul's Cathedral built in the 16th Century and observed the crowds in the theatre district known as Picadilly Circus. London is the personification of history. How Hitler could have bombed this city is unbelievable. It was certainly not a military target and bombing it was totally unnecessary.

The Thames River empties into the English Channel. The many bridges which cross it are very low and consist of multiple arches. There are ships in this river which are much higher than the bridges. How did they get there, and how do they get through the bridges to the ocean?

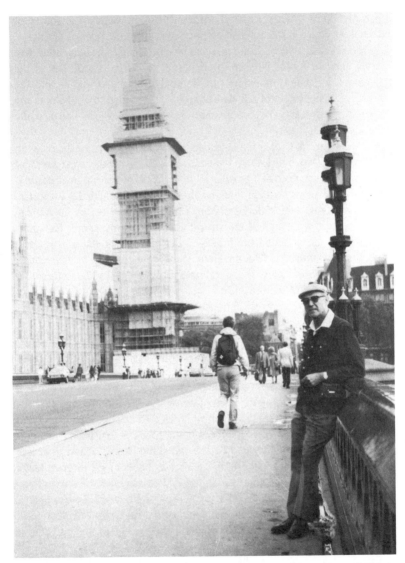

The clock, BIG BEN was being overhauled as I paused on the Westminster Bridge in London.

The tide is the answer, plus smoke stacks that fold down towards the deck. Half the day water flows from the ocean up the Thames, and the other half it flows down the Thames. When it flows up, the water is salty. When it flows towards the ocean it loses its salinity. London uses the upper portion of this river as its source of drinking water. The source of the Thames River is the English countryside plus underground springs.

After a brief taste of London I boarded a Sabena Jet and after five hours landed in Kano, Nigeria, to refuel. I was able to walk out of the plane door for a few moments "to smell the air of Africa" I told the stewardess. The middle of Africa was so hot, I was glad to get back to my air-conditioned seat. The countryside appeared rather desolate and the ground parched.

From the air the Camaroon landscape appeared to be a vast forest, with many rivers. Two hours later I landed in Douala on the west coast of Africa where I changed to a smaller jet which flew me to my final destination, Yaounde, a city which does not have a large enough Jet airport to land the super jet which flew me from London. I was met by an African youth who held up a sign at the airport spelling out my name. He spoke only French. He gathered my luggage, and after about the 4th passport inspection he deposited me at the Hotel Des Deputies, very well air conditioned. He was to return in 30 minutes to take me to the seminar of students for a day of lectures.

My room was all right by European standards. My main concern was the efficiency of the air conditioning since I was in the very midst of the blistering tropics of Equatorial Africa. The Congo borders the Camaroons. I sat in the hotel's lobby waiting for my chauffer to return. He wore a uniform with an American flag insignia on his shirt that said "U.S. Aid Mission", the State Department branch that pays for this mission that I'm on to teach Africans the intricacies of conscious sedation anesthesia.

An hour went by—he did not return. I tried to call the Aid Mission. I tried to call the three phone numbers I was given at JHPIEGO in Baltimore, but there was no answer. I finally called the U.S. Embassy. The line was busy for three hours. Not until 4 P.M. was I able to get through to the U.S. Embassy. They switched me to the Aid Mission who knew nothing about my arrival. "Who did you say you are?" I shouted "Shane, Shane, I've been here all day and the students are waiting for my lectures." "What lectures?" I was so exasperated I was ready to fly out of this poverty-stricken rear end of the earth.

Finally at 4:30 they sent the same chauffer to pick me up. He took me to George Vishio who was in charge of the Aid Mission for the U.S. The lack of responsibility and organization here was appalling.

This man had no idea of when I was to lecture, or where, or in which hospital I was to instruct the Africans in conscious sedation. "We will decide all this tomorrow," he said. He then introduced me to Dr. Richard

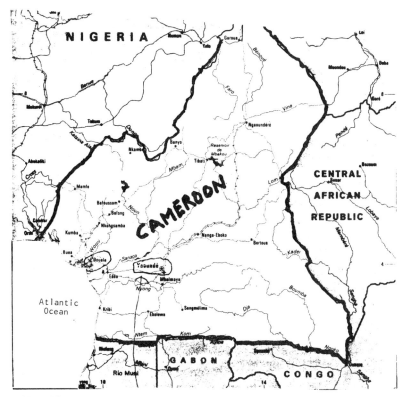

Map of Cameroon, the official names is: United Republic of Cameroon. It is located on the west coast of central Africa.

Schutz, a physician from Frankfurt, Germany, who is the anesthesiologist in charge of the Central Hospital in Yaounde. Schutz is spending two years here as part of a contract to some religious mission. He has one more year to serve and can't wait till the year is up. Schutz took me in hand, and took me through every nook and crany of this hospital. There are only two in the city. I spend four hours with him, till night fall. Then he drove me to my hotel.

What I am about to reveal I would never believe if I read it somewhere. I would think the writer was simply prejudiced. But what I saw, I saw, and I'm about to describe the way it was, just as I saw it, eye-witnessed.

Before I tell of the state of medical care in this country I must describe the status of mankind here.

Poverty is a poorly descriptive word. It does not convey the lassitude,

the hopelessness, the malnutrition, the futureless future of these miserable, black people, who look exactly like the blacks in Baltimore, New
York and Detroit. Their main diet consists of bananas, peanuts and a large
tuber which resembles a potato. Meat, cheese, canned goods, and even
bread are for the few who have government positions, and they are only a
slight rung above the poverty-stricken.

There are two supermarkets in the city, one known as Score and the
other Prisunic. Score is owned by a Greek. These supermarkets resemble
the A & P, but who patronizes them? The few government workers and the
whites who are living here to help exploit the oil and other minerals as the
masses buy their food right off the food venders on the streets and along
the roadways where bananas and apples are piled high wherever you turn,
not on carts or platforms but right on the dirt pathways that serve as
sidewalks.

The atmosphere of the city reeks of a burning charcoal odor reminiscent of India's cities, Calcutta, Bombay and New Delhi.

Men display their manhood by the number of children they claim from
a multitude of women. This is the macho culture. There are no Mercedes
or mansions, or jewelry or swimming pools to proclaim their achievements, just teeming crowds of babies and children.

But what kind of a culture can it be when syphilis, gonorrhea, and Aids
are so rampant that the public health service, if you can call it that, will
not treat these public scourges unless the victims buy drugs such as penicillin themselves from a pharmacy, an expense they can't afford. And
there's no hope at all for the Aids sufferers.

Tuberculosis is rampant because of malnutrition and the close, packed-
in living quarters consisting mostly of tin roof hovels.

If an accident occurs at night you're as good as dead. No doctor will
see you after 5 P.M. You just bleed out till morning. Broken bones remain
unattended till morning, if the surgeon ever decides to show up. Fractured
hips and femurs are not operated with modern pinning procedures because
the orthopedic pins cost too much. All the world uses disposable plastic
syringes to inject medicines since it is difficult to sterilize a syringe.
Boiling a syringe does *not* kill viruses such as herpes, T.B., tetanus, and
Aids. The syringes in two hospitals here are *boiled!* I saw patients dying
from tetanus.

It is really very frightening to be here should a serious medical problem
arise in myself.

Transurethral prostatectomies are unknown. Should a man's urine
block up they rip out his prostate through an abdominal incision and most

of these patients die of infection, especially if the family cannot buy the sulfa or penicillin to treat the patient because the hospitals do not supply medications. The surgeon writes a prescription and the family must go to a pharmacy and bring the medicine to the nurse or doctor who will then inject it via a non-sterile syringe. If I hadn't seen all this I would never believe it.

The seriousness of all this is that the doctors do not care for their black brothers. There is no camaraderie in misfortune here. The Arabs and Moslems have some hope in misfortune. They are happy in illness because they may more quickly be in the arms of Allah and paradise. But what hope is there for these descendants of Ham?

The interior of the central hospital which is a series of one-story buildings housing its 200 beds, spreads over a large courtyard. If you saw what I witnessed you would have vomited. I saw a ward with 20 beds, an intensive-care ward with post-surgical patients, lying on army cots, separated by one foot of space. No privacy, no curtains between, men and women intermixed including children, with abscesses draining, tuberculosis rampant, open wounds, hepatitis, pneumonia. There was no available oxygen, no respirators for those finding it difficult to breath, only one EKG machine in the entire hospital and that was broken. An X-ray costs $25.00 and if the patient can't pay for it, it won't be taken, and few to none of the patients can pay it.

The one surgeon who can perform prostatectomies charges the astronomical sum of $600 or else you get a catheter in your bladder through an abdominal incision to relieve the urinary backup and simply die of infection.

The neurosurgeon hasn't opened a head or operated on a brain in years. He says he hasn't found it necessary. The patients simply die and he couldn't care less.

Such indifference to suffering was unbelievable.

And the dirt and filth in the wards was appalling. Paint was peeling off the ceilings, sandy dirt was on the floors since the grounds around the buildings are unpaved and muddy. I walked into the operating rooms with my street clothes on, an unheard of event in U.S. hospitals. Sometimes the water supply stops for two or three days at a time. Drinking water is kept in a 50-gallon oil drum and is ladled out as needed. It was full of dirt particles when I examined it.

The delivery rooms were a series of four, iron tables, *without* mattresses. Women were lying there pushing babies out with no professional help in attendance, only disinterested, bored, black women called nurses, sitting around knitting. There was no equipment for resusitating babies, who are born with impaired breathing. They just die. And the infant death rate is tremendous. Acute appendicitis here is a death warrant. So is an abscessed tooth. I saw pregnant girls, teenagers, in labor lying on a wooden bench out on the walkways; there was no room in the delivery room. Filth was so widespread and nauseating that I seriously thought of getting the hell out of this garbage can of a city.

With conscious sedation requiring the establishment of an empathetic rapport between the anesthetist and the patient, how can this ever be accomplished when the surgeons and anesthetists are so indifferent to death and suffering among their own people, so indifferent to the filth, to the lack of sterility, and especially to the indifference as to whether or not a relative will go out and buy penicillin in some pharmacy for a child, wife, or husband who is dying with high fever from infection?

The death rate in the hospitals from neglect and infection is an absolute scandal.

But there is a new modern building housing the Ministry of Health. What a laugh!! The health officials sit in their air-conditioned, new offices administering a health program that resembles the hospital abattoirs of the 18th century in Paris before the concept of sepsis was understood.

I could now begin to comprehend why there was no organized program for my arrival here, despite the effort and arrangements made by JHPIEGO in Baltimore a month before I left.

There is a medical laboratory here that does all the tests on blood, feces, sputum, pus, etc. to help in diagnosis. Dr. Shutz cannot depend on the hospital's laboratory doing the tests. They are either not done, results are lost, or he never receives the reports. This is run by blacks. He sends his specimens to an independently run French lab. It's inconvenient, but the contrast is obvious. One would think that the ministers of health (George Vishio is one of them) would be embarrassed at this indicting, damaging contrast. But who cares? Black lives are cheap. And the blacks themselves are too apathetic to demand better treatment.

When I see what goes on in the rest of the world with regard to food, water supply, education, medical care and human welfare I'm glad I live in the U S of A as Archie Bunker says.

There is one other hospital in the city of Yaounde, a partly-private hospital, private for those who can pay, such as government officials and a handful of the wealthy class. It's called the University Hospital. The difference between this and the public welfare hospital known as the Central Hospital, is the difference between morning and late P.M., not night. It's

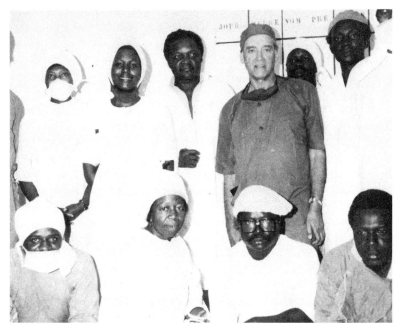

The operating room staff at the University Hospital in the Cameroons. The author is fourth from left.

modern and clean, but already the signs of apathy and deterioration are setting in. They wanted me to work in both hospitals but I refused to even enter the horrible Central Welfare Hospital. I was actually fearful for my own safety, but I did teach at the University Hospital.

The black people administering the JHPIEGO funds here, are totally incomprehensible. There is no organization, no planning, no meaning to time or schedule. I finally met the group I was to train for the first time three days after I arrived. I sat in my hotel room reading, as there was nothing else to do. The streets here are without sidewalks. People walk in mud. I had no desire to even explore this jungle, much less walk the streets. The hotel I was in was rather new but there were ants and bugs in my room. I had the room changed to one that was just "sanitized". I found the same ants and bugs plus mice. These pests are probably immune to chemical sprays. What I am doing may sound glamorous but it is not. It is certainly no vacation. I met some young jean-clad chaps, all excited about being here. They're here for the Peace Corps for two years, and they are not being housed in the 1st class hotel I'm in, not even a 4th class hotel. Can you imagine the vermin and bugs with which they'll be confronted.

When I met my group of over 30 people among whom were anesthesiologists, nurse anesthetists, and gynecologists, they sat there very immobile and expressionless and appeared dull as if they did not know what I was talking about.

It's peculiar sitting here in my room all day. I feel as if I'm in prison. There's no way I can escape from here unless the airline books me on an earlier flight out of here. Think of these poverty-stricken natives who in their lifetimes would never be able to buy a plane ticket, and where would they go without money? I suppose you have to see this part of the world to appreciate the absolute luxurious life we have in the U.S.

I finished reading TRIPLE by Ken Follett, an unreal spy saga. It was perfect reading for this enforced isolation and idleness.

Now for some facts about the Cameroon. This country is about the size of California, and houses $8^{1}/_{2}$ million black people. There are 200 ethnic tribes here with various African religions including Islam and Christianity. There are 24 different African languages but French is the official language with English second. Education is *not* compulsory. Only one half the population can read and the average length of life is 47 years. Agriculture is the main source of income for 83 per cent of the people who are engaged in it.

They export cocoa, coffee, tropical wood, oil, and iron ore. Because of this kind of trade the U.S. maintains a large embassy here with a contingent of marines. Texaco, Mobil Oil, and Shell, IBM are all well represented here. I saw Israeli canned goods in one of the grocery stores.

About 20,000 Europeans and 800 U.S. citizens live here. There is a University of Yaounde that offers courses in English and French. The University Hospital (the fancy one) is part of the Medical School. This University was established in 1961.

Much of the slave trade originated here and the blacks resemble the negroes in the U.S.

Cameroon history in the modern sense began in 1884, when Germany, Britain and France all attempted to annex the country. The Germans controlled it first. Then after World War I the country was divided between Britain and France and run by them under a League of Nations mandate. After world War II Britain and France ruled here under "trusteeships". In 1958, Cameroon achieved independence under the U.N. General Assembly just as Israel did in 1948.

The president is a black named Paul Biya; the prime minister is

Maigari Bouba and other officials have similar unpronounceable names. There are 9,000 soldiers in the Army. The U.S. pours 1$^1/_2$ million each year to finance the Cameroon Army. Why? Ask Texaco. The U.S. also pays for the AID (Agency for International Development) that pays my expenses and that of the Peace Corp Volunteers.

Without a map of Africa one would never have a concept of where he is in relationship with the rest of the world. You board a plane in London, in seconds you are above the clouds and the blue heavens above are identical around the earth. You sit in the plane for seven hours, eat, read, watch a movie, soon your ears feel as if they might burst and the pilot announces you are about to land in Kano, Nigeria. You descend out of the clouds and all you see are a vast expanse of green trees in a rain forest. The plane lands. All airports look alike everywhere—even the Ben Gurion in Israel looks like the ones in Africa and Paris and in Baltimore. The plane takes on fuel. In seconds you are above the clouds again and the blue above. An hour later you descend beneath the clouds and there are the same brown patches of farm land and batches of trees seen over Maryland, and the pilot announces we are about to land in Duala, the 2nd largest city in Cameroon.

Travellers in the future will never come to this part of the world by foot or horse or camel anymore. Those who travelled by animal or foot understand distances. By air there is simply no comprehension. Without a map of Africa I could be in the midst of Baltimore's Druid Hill Park. I wonder sometimes if it is better to be in the 4th grade and fantasize about the adventure and excitement of some day going to such far away places as the Congo, Cameroon, Nigeria, Zanzibar, rather than be here and have all your adventurous dreams exploded by the filth, mud, mosquitos, ants, and bugs which permeate even the most modern hotels. Imagine what it's like in the hovels and shacks with tin roofs, no running water and no toilets which house the majority of inhabitants of these so-called adventurous outposts such as Cameroon, Congo, Tunisia, Morocco, Egypt, India, Calcutta, and Indonesia.

In grammar and high school few of the teachers could ever afford such extensive travel as I have experienced and probably labor under the same false illusions regarding far away places as do their 4th grade students. The teachers therefore augment these fantasies. I can well remember my 4th grade fantasies. Now they are all gone, disintegrated by the truth of reality.

The great masses of the poverty-stricken who inhabit these 3rd world nations are under no tension and misery because of their primitive environment. The human being has a built in mechanism that evades this potential problem. It is called adaptability. A child born here amidst flies, roaches, rats and the smell of sewers adapts to it. This is normal for him. There is no other environment with which to compare it. He's happy as he grows up. He even becomes immune to the surrounding infection inherent in the drinking water and the fleas carried by rats. But I have to drink Perrier water and fear to go out of the hotel after dusk because of the malaria-carrying mosquitos. I won't even eat in the hotel dining room since the food is handled by tuberculous cooks and waiters and is used as a landing strip by flies and other vermin.

Food is a real inconvenience for me. I keep in my room many bottles of Perrier water. This is imported from France. They have Cameroon mineral water in bottles at half the price. But I saw how they bottle mineral water in Puerto Vallarta, Mexico. Local water with a "mineral water" label. I have cans of sardines, tuna, an immersible electric water heater, peanuts, and a box of prunes and raisins and a can of Inka, also peelable fruit which I wash in soap and water, then rinse in whiskey before I eat the "peeled" fruit. Who in the hell wants to live like this? Imagine the American Ambassador who lives here with his wife and children. There is no structure here impervious to the swarms of vermin inherent in this tropical, equatorial rectum of the earth.

I ran out of fruit yesterday. I decided to order some from the real fancy dining room in the hotel. On the menu it is listed as "Basket of Fresh Fruit". I sat at a table and ordered it. They brought me a large tray with a whole pineapple, uncut, in the center and surrounded by tiny tangerines, dirty looking oranges and speckled apples. All were wet, as if washed. I could not have the pineapple, that was for decoration. I selected the oranges, apples and tangerines. The dirt on my hands from simply picking up this wet fruit was unbelievable.

I wiped off the dirt with my napkin, then wrapped it all in another napkin and took it to my room for more intensive treatment.

In other rooms in this first class hotel some guests complained of mice as well as roaches, big ones.

I finally got my ticket changed. The irresponsible doctor who was to have arranged my program here has a sister who works in the Cameroon Airline ticket office. She changed my reservation so I could leave this hellhole one week earlier. I told the doctor I had to leave a week earlier than I contracted for and could not meet the 2nd group of students 200 miles north of here because my stomach was giving me problems.

A week after arriving I checked out of the Hotel Des Deputies, went to the Yaounde Airport. The bedlam here was unbelievable. There was no organization. The airport was running with roaches. The little stand which sold coffee hadn't been cleaned in years. The lines of pushing, shoving, squeezing, screeching blacks was so unreal that if I took motion pictures of the bedlam one would think it was set up as a comic act. Imagine having to open your luggage at a Baltimore airline ticket counter while you stand in the packed line like sardines for inspection prior to flying the short distance to New York. It was not the carry-on hand luggage, but my major, heavy luggage. How was I to get to it. Where was I to lay it out to open it with everyone stampeding over, around, and on top of me? Then an apathetic, bored native, in army fatigues, with a gun holster, ran his fingers through my luggage, picked up my multiple bottles of Vitamin C I'm bringing to my daughter Nancy in Israel and queries me in French— "Que es'que Cette"?—(what's this?) "Small atom bombs to blow Yaounde off the map," I told him in English. And everyone had to go through this nonsense. After one receives a boarding pass he gets his hand luggage inspected. This is another long line of delay. By this time the plane is already 40 minutes delayed on take off because of this totally disorganized, incomprehensible, inefficiency. Also, there's no air conditioning, everyone is sweating. The room is small and the odor is nauseating.

Finally, I somehow got on the plane, an old Boeing 737, but piloted by a French pilot. This was a short flight of 100 miles to Duala where I changed to a Jumbo Jet for the seven-hour flight to Paris. How clean and beautiful the blue heavens looked after the fiasco of Yaounde.

Here are some interesting aspects of Black culture in this African nation:

Polygamy is legal here. My A.I.D. driver, Pierre,is the child of his father's 3rd wife. His father has 4 wives and 28 children.

He told me that when a man chooses his 2nd, 3rd, 4th and 10th wife, he must provide a separate hut for each wife. In the case of his father, who owns a farm, he spends one week with each wife. During that week she cooks his meals and takes care of him. Then she doesn't see him for 3 weeks while he's with the other wives. Pierre told me the trouble begins when he tells wife #1 and wife #2 that he now wants a third wife. This invariably causes strife. If any of the wives want to leave, they automatically lose the children. The father has title to them. The children are extra laboring hands on the farm, as well as the wife.

One head of a village not far from Yaounde has 27 wives and over 210 children. He spends one night with each wife. But women can have only *one* husband. This is the way society was laid out in the Old Testament, the Torah. And these natives never heard of the Torah. Marriage is a civil affair. The man and gal go to the "Bureau", sign up and they're married. It is the same for divorce. But the man always gets the children. Women's lib is unknown here. Abortion is illegal, officially. But if one pays the gynecologist $100 he will abort in the University Hospital and give a psychiatric excuse to circumvent the law. They'll be using conscious sedation to do this in the future if my instruction ever sinks in.

Young girls who can't afford the price, go to an illegal nurse abortionist who performs it for $25 in a dirty, metal-roofed hovel where she lives, and most of these patients go home and die in several days from infection. Those girls who are not married and become pregnant have their babies and drop them in the nearest garbage can, in an area remote from where they live. This is common practice here so as not to disgrace their mothers. (They hardly know their fathers.)

One of the major problems here is gonorrhea. This disease causes P.I.D. or pelvic inflammatory disease. This causes adhesions in the fallopian tubes and renders the girls sterile. It is a birth-controlling disease to prevent overpopulation, but it does cause severe pelvic pain for long periods of time.

Contraceptives are illegal, but they may be obtained, only on prescription from a physician. Of course, it is necessary to pay the physician before he gives the prescription. Since this is expensive and complicated one may have to spend half a day waiting to see the physician plus his fee; there, it's simpler to make love without protection. As a consequence syphilis, gonorrhea and AIDS spread here like a prairie fire.

When I met my students and demonstrated conscious sedation in the University Hospital they forgot to supply an interpreter. This was to be expected since they didn't even know I was being sent. The interpreter I had happened to be a gynecologist who trained at Howard University in Washington and he spoke French and English fluently. He did a great job. Without him the entire session might have been wasted. French for "Do Not Move" is "Ne Bougez Pas" and French for "Do Not Say Ooh Ooh" is "Ne Dit Pas Ooh Ooh".

I had to remind the patients under conscious sedation not to move and not to say oooh oooh. The patients got off the operating table themselves and walked back to their ward. It was quite impressive.

In the operating room the professor of gynecology posed a question: "Dr. Shane, you are using five drugs to produce this state of conscious sedation. We are sedating patients with only two drugs—Valium and Demerol. Why should we use five instead of two?"

I said, "Your patients with two drugs are so knocked out, practically unconscious, that it requires four orderlies to lift them off the operating table since they cannot move. Furthermore, back in their ward their tongues may fall back and they may die of asphyxiation. My patients who receive small quantities of five drugs get off the operating table themselves, walk back to the ward on their own power and eat lunch. That's why five small doses are better than two big doses. It's safer. This slow thinking physician had to think about this before he concluded it was safer and more logical.

I travelled 1st class from Duala in the Cameroons to Paris.

PARIS

I checked in at the Astra Hotel located at 29 Rue Coumartin near the Rue De L'Opera.

The plane ride at 37,000 feet was uneventful and all I could see from the window was brownish-red earth, the burning hot sands of the Sahara Desert far below, roasting in a glittering haze. It was as though there was no intervening stretch of Africa or the Mediterranean between the Cameroon and Paris. Only a French film, caviar, much wine and excellent camaraderie between myself and the passenger seated next to me who was a 747 Boeing pilot on vacation.

I spent Saturday walking the streets of Paris which I love to do. I walked along the Seine to the Austerlitz Railroad Station and back via the Rue de Rivoli. I had wine, cheese and bread sent to my room and promptly fell asleep from the wine. I had walked about 10 miles.

The next day I decided to view the French countryside to the west of Paris. I boarded a train en route to Bordeaux but remained on the train for half the journey and disembarked at the city of Angers, the first stop after Le Mans, remained in Angers for a few hours, then returned to Paris.

The countryside was flat, interspersed with farms growing corn and wheat and grazing milk cows. The railroad line, as are all lines in France, are electrified.

The ride to Angers, to the west of Paris, was 125 miles. I walked through the town which was like sections of Paris.

Some of the towns through which the train passed are Chartres, Le

Mans, Sable, Champaign, Rennes, La Suze, Voivre, La Loupe, Maintenon, Epernon, Le Perray, San Quentin, and Rive Gouch.

The flatness of the ground and the surrounding countryside resembled the Eastern shore of Maryland, and parts of Nebraska. Because it was Sunday it appeared from the train that the towns were asleep. But the sidewalk cafes in Angers were all crowded with the residents eating their Sunday dinners out on the sidewalk.

There is a peculiarly-shaped freight car on the sidings of Europe. These are seen especially in Germany and Austria, but one also sees them in France, Poland, Czeckoslovakia and other countries. They have a rounded roof and a single sliding door. There are only two wheels on each side of the car, one in front, one in back and they appear to have spokes. These freight cars, I call "Juden Cars" because it was these cars which Hitler loaded with Jews on the way to the ovens of Auschwitz. Those destined to perish, and there were 6 million, were loaded into these cars, standing up, and squeezed and packed in so that no one could move and had to stand erect, sometimes for days, until the trains reached Auschwitz. Many died standing, and the stink from urine and feces when the sealed doors were opened was unbearable. When the "passengers" were told to undress and proceed to the "shower rooms" one can imagine the enthusiasm of such a treat. Little did they know that Cyclone "B", the deadly cyanide gas would be emitted from the shower heads. I remember these cars from my experience in Auschwitz, Poland in 1948. And the sight of them in France evokes once again, those sad, depressing memories of almost 40 years ago which I described in the book AS I SAW IT. It seems these "Juden Cars" are still popular in France and in Europe. When I see them standing alone on a siding in the freight yard where the train stops in a town, my otherwise cheerful, enlightened mood, becomes melancholy and introspective. It was from all of these towns that Hitler gathered the Jews in these two-wheeled freight cars for their long ride of death, and the truth of this never leaves my memory.

I returned to Paris at about 4 P.M. and walked from the Montparnas Station to the Place de la Concord where the great Egyptian obelisk reigns supreme with the Arc d'Triumph at the opposite end of the Champs D'Elysees. But I could go no further. The streets across the Concorde were blocked by 1,000 police to permit a great European event to occur—the all-Europe Bicycle Race which was ending at this point. There were thousands of people all cheering the Parisian cyclist. It was like an Oriole World Series event and I couldn't care less; in fact, I couldn't even get to my hotel.

When the event was finally over I sat at an outdoor cafe on the Blvd. Haussmann, known as Triadov Haussmann and drank a large pitcher of beer. It was hot and thirst was overwhelming. This cafe was located at the corner of Rue de Rome, right in front of Au Printemps, the big department store on Boulevard Haussmann near the Rue De L'opera.

Paris today belongs to the youth. The older people seem so out of place mainly because there are so many young people crowding the streets. Brassieres are out. The natural floppy breast look is in. It seems that jeans are now out. What they're wearing, and "they" means the females, is a white operating-room, pair of white pants, baggy, that goes as far as the ankles. The peculiar style, seems to spread so quickly in Europe and America.

But the city itself is so unusual, so international, so cosmopolitan. The buildings usually have imprinted on the second stories the name and date of the designing architect. The dates are usually between 1890 and 1910. The intricate iron work on the upper-window balconies is seen nowhere else in the world. The beautiful rococo carvings on the most inauspicious buildings is just amazing by today's square, plain, modern, ugly buildings. The city is flowing with a hundred different tour buses. I think George Gershwin really captured the essence of the place in his music An American in Paris.

I thought how wonderful it is to be once again in civilization and out of the deep darkness of Africa. It takes a trip like this for one to count his blessings, and especially the blessings inherent in the United States despite the Reagans, the Klu Klux Klan, and all the false TV advertising. After observing every continent and every capital city, I agree with Archie Bunker: give me the good old U.S. of A. To understand this one must travel widely with open eyes and not with blinkers.

This Paris is a city beyond descriptive words. It breaths, pulsates, reverberates and shouts history. The United States and all its cities are so young by comparison that a trip to Paris simply overwhelms; and every time I come here I am overwhelmed.

Paris was founded before Jesus was born, over 2300 years ago. There is a cemetery here known as Cemetiere Montmartre with the oddest-looking tomb stones. Buried here are famous composers like Berlioz, and Offenbach and authors like Alexander Dumas and Stendhal. There's an immense building with Greek columns resembling the Pantheon in Athens, and the name of it here in Paris is also the Pantheon. It is the burial place of only great men. Some of those buried in its walls are Emile Zola, Victor Hugo, and Jacque Rousseau.

Victor Hugo who wrote The Hunchback of Notre Dame in the late 1900's was responsible for bringing the Notre Dame Cathedral to the attention of the world. This famous piece of architecture, built in the 13th century was deteriorating by the 19th Century. The Hunchback of Notre Dame was so famous a book, that it sparked a restitution movement to replace and refinish every carving that was deteriorating, including the roof, the steeples, and the ugly gargoyles overhanging the spires.

At the Arc D'Triumph, commenced in 1806 by Napoleon and completed in 1836 after Napoleon's death, there is an eternal flame burning to commemorate those who died in both World Wars. Everyday a bouquet of flowers is placed near the flame by the military.

Napoleon is buried in a special building occupying a city clock called the Hotel Des Invalides. The word, "Hotel" is used to mean either "great mansion" or "hospital". In fact it was a hospital for invalids, but it was converted into an appropriate burial place to memorialize Napoleon. Another military man is also buried there—Marshall Foch of World War I fame.

The spot where the Arc D'Triumph is located is known as the Etoile which means "Star". This is appropriate since 12 Avenues radiate from this "Etoile". One famous one is the Champs Elysees. On the other side of the Arc it is called the Avenue of the Grand Armee. Another Avenue is named Foch. It is on Avenue Foch that the world's millionaires like the Prince of Monoco and the Rothchilds have their apartment mansions. But they are not individual homes. The buildings all run together with no division between them, like immensely long five story row houses with no front porches!

The street names in Paris are for the most part names memorializing famous individuals such as: Rue Alexis Carrel, Rue August Compte, Rue Voltaire, or Avenue President Kennedy. The Avenue Victor Hugo is one of the 12 Avenues that radiate from the Arc D'Triumph.

On a high hill overlooking all of Paris, like Mt. Scopus overlooks Jerusalem, there is a basilica known as the Basilique Du Sacre Coeur— translated means the Church of the Sacred Heart (of Jesus). It is located at a section known as Montmartre which means the Mt. of Martyrs. The Romans who occupied Paris before Jesus, built a temple there and called it the Mt. of Mercury to honor their god Mercury who had wings on his heels. It is now renamed Montmartre. The interesting aspect of this high point in Paris is not only the breathtaking view, as from an airplane, but famous artists work here. There is a small square where they all congregate and paint. The place is brimming over with tourists who come to buy their paintings and have their own faces produced in charcoal and pen and ink. They are really outstanding artists, not the kind you see at an amusement park or a circus.

Most of the people who work in Paris live in the western suburbs and get there via the Gare St. Lazar, the St. Lazare Railroad station. It's similar to the Long Island Railroad which transports thousands to New York City each day.

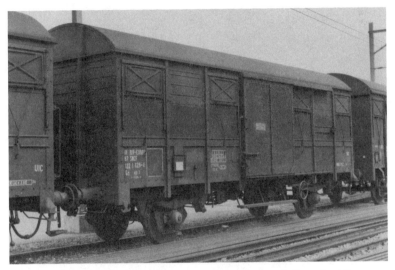

"Juden Cars." These are the freight cars, seen in railroad yards throughout Europe, which the nazis used to transport Jews to the ovens in Auschwitz.

CHAPTER IV

THE SEARCH FOR TRUTH

I am sometimes strangulated in the creative process by my appalling vanity. In attempting to set forth on paper those primitive wonderous thought processes which tell us of the Creator the Universe, I find myself thinking of what someone else will think of what I am writing and almost immediately it hampers the free flow of what I inwardly feel. If only I could put into words that intimate, inward knowledge which so infrequently suffuses through my mind during rare moments of contemplation, as when I behold in a quiet world, the last bright star at the birth of dawn, or listen to the ocean's incessant motion as it licks a concrete seawall. I thought of the sun just below the horizon, a fixed point in space, while the point which I occupied on earth was slowly turning to meet it. I saw the dome of sky meet the sea and as I turned from left to right, no more perfect circle could man imagine than the one created on the horizon's edge. I thought of the universe before light was created and wondered if G-d too disliked the inkiness of darkness. But here again I interject my own vanity and attempt to ascribe to G-d those whimsical feelings which only man can feel. It is profoundly difficult to imagine a substance not of matter; to imagine a Creator not of substance. The contemplation of infinite space, of soaring off into an infinity that is forever without end makes me for a moment forget my vanity as I tremble in helplessness.

One needs only to behold the sun, a commonplace object, with us every day, the source of light. It is so commonplace that rarely in our lives do we think of it except that we hope it will shine when we plan a picnic or travel to the seashore. But this sun, this incomprehensible ball of nuclear fission, never goes out; it never loses its brilliance; it never cools off. Without it there could be no rain, no bread, no life. It is of equal importance to the sustenance of the life of man as is the oxygen concentration of the atmosphere which never varies.

Aside from the hidden mysteries of the universe I need only contemplate the sun to achieve that inner knowledge of God's existence. For the sun just simply did not happen by itself.

Regardless of the atheist's logical deception, or of the scientists' mathematical vanity, the sure inner knowledge of G-d's presence will ultimately make men reach out from deep within to touch, for a fleeting moment, that evanescent filament of eternity and to sense Paul Tillich's ultimate concern.

BELIEFS

Everyone has a belief in some force that rules the universe over which he has little control. Some believe in science, some in communism, some in agnosticism (which means "show me" and prove it to my eyesight if you want me to believe it). Some believe in "Nature", some believe in Jesus, some like Buddhist and Hindus believe in idols, and some believe in G-d. Those who do not believe in the G-d of the Old Testament prefer to call their god science, or communism, or Jesus, or nature.

This chapter will reveal how my beliefs evolved and why. One of my objectives in life was the search for truth, a very elusive concept, and one that is difficult to ascertain. I searched for truth in advertising and found it constantly faulty and misleading. For example, the advertisement for Fleishman's Margarine, reads: "Made of 100% corn oil; eat it to reduce cholesterol." True it does consist of 100% corn oil, but what the advertisement does not tell is that most of the corn oil is hydrogenated (which makes it solid and not liquid) and that this alteration of the corn oil by bubbling hydrogen through it is a greater factor in causing heart attacks than butter or animal fat. A half truth is more misleading than a full lie, and most advertising seen in newspapers, magazines and TV consist of half truths.

The advertising on all hot dog packages state "these hot dogs are 100% beef." True they do consist of 100% beef, but the advertisement indulges in a half truth. It does not tell us that 95% of the hot dog is not beef meat, but beef fat which is poison to the coronary arteries of human beings. And kosher hot dogs contain the same high content of beef fat as non-kosher hot dogs, so they are no better.

We are bombarded with half truths that emanate from our national government as exemplified by the Johnson and Nixon administrations in promoting the ridiculous wars in Vietnam and Korea and now the Reagan administration in Nicaragua and by the evening TV molders of public opinion in the United States such as Dan Rather on CBS, Peter Jennings on ABC, and Tom Brokaw on NBC. These men know the truth of what's going on, but can reveal only half of it (a half truth) if they want to retain their jobs. The full truth of the rivalry between the USSR and the US is that the US must have a perpetual enemy on the horizon, ever ready to attack us, if we are to justify the billions of dollars paid out annually to military contractors for atomic bombs, soldier's shoe laces, military bombers, soldier's socks and toilet paper, everything military from the sublime to the ridiculous. And the majority of the military expenditures is for planes and tanks and bombs that rapidly become obsolescent. New models of bombs and guns appear yearly. The obsolescent material must be dumped in the ocean to make way for new military contracts. We must remain up-to-date if we are to keep up with the artificially-created enemy, the Russians.

A few years ago we were friendly with the Russians and we created an oriental enemy in the Chinese. During the McCarthy era the Chinese were going to overrun California and, especially, San Francisco. Now the Chinese are our friends and the new, more-formidable enemy is the Soviet Union. Therefore we must spend 230 billion dollars for "Star Wars" to contain that vicious tiger, to protect our freedom. Every scientist of note in the world has denounced the stupidity of "Star Wars" as a military boon-doggle, to keep the military industrial factories busy in the United States.

Some believe that if we do not give these billions of tax dollars to the military industrialists we will see an overwhelming rise in unemployment and the same expenditure of billions will be paid out in welfare checks to the unemployed.

This may be so. The point I am making is that there was half truth inherent in the "Star Wars" military expenditure of the Reagan administration and the failure of the Reykjavik Summit that could have meant a world free of atomic bombs. In addition, there was a lack of full reporting this aspect of it by the ABC, CBS, and NBC anchormen who mislead American public opinion every night on TV throughout the U.S.A. at 7 & 11 P.M.

So much for half truths, and the lack of truth in advertising, newscasting, and government.

I have also searched for truth in the concept of evolution as taught in our universities, and whether or not our religious beliefs, Jewish or Christian and Islamic are based on truth or shrouded in myth.

There isn't a university professor in the U.S. who would risk his academic stature and standing among his peers, by stating that there is not one shred of evidence to uphold the theory of evolution which is taught in many institutions not as a theory, but as fact.

The following is an exerpt from the writings of an electrical engineer named Robert Perlman who summed up the falsity and the half truth in teaching evolution as law or fact, instead of the theory which it is. I am quoting this at length since Perlman expressed it so well:*

"Every intelligent individual looks at himself and at the world and ponders the question—Where do we and our world come from? Science answers "evolution" which has been the basis of modern thought. The basic statement of evolution is: "Out of the primeval ooze arose life. The animals gradually changed and the fittest of the new species were selected by the struggle for existence. Every bigger, better, more complex species were thus formed by the struggle, creating all nature, and man himself, among whom the struggle continues that selects the fittest and will produce superior races of superman. This is progress."

This is also one of the biggest frauds ever perpetrated by intelligent men on mankind. Evolution is a theory without proof of any kind and it is, to this day, taught in our universities as a fact. It is indoctrinated everywhere from kindergarten to the PhD. candidate. No scientist dares question it without losing his academic standing. Why this massive acceptance of a fraud?

Here's what the evolutionists say is proof. They show a similarity among different species in their appearance, skeletons, and embryos. This is true. The biology books and encyclopedias all exhibit the classical paintings of how man emerged from the lowest organism in the sea, how he emerged from the sea, learned to breath, then walk as an ape who later evolved into a man. The paintings are the pure imagination of a skilled artist.

These so called proofs are made by biologists. A biologist is one who studies and classifies animals by their internal and external appearance. The key word here is appearance, and all their proofs are based on appearance. And if one is to base the proof of evolution on appearance, such as the biology book paintings portray, it is fraudulent to teach this as a truth or fact. The truth of evolution must be based not on appearance but on FUNCTION or action. The color, and size of bones as depicted in the encyclopedia are superficial. The

*Robert Perlman: Science vs Evolution. A chapter in A Science and Torah Reader, a publication of Jewish Youth Monthly; published by U.O.J.C. New York, 1970.

question of evolution cannot be decided by showing that animals can change superficially, but only by determining whether they can evolve FUNCTIONALLY, by changing their basic designs and grow new organs.

The electric eel will serve as an example of function. In the eel family there are eels with electricity and eels without electricity. They both have survived to this day. One third of the electric eel is an electric powerhouse, having more than 5000 batteries and turning out, at the eels command, a 500 volt high powered shock to thwart its enemies. This voltage is 5 times as strong as the electricity that lights our homes. It will paralyze a man or another fish.

Now how did this eel, an ordinary eel, invent and design an electric powerhouse with insulation, switches, etc? If evolution is operating here it must start with one battery. This amount of electricity would not even harm a minnow. The eel must then take this utterly useless equipment and add hundreds of batteries, electrically and correctly wired, before it reaches a point where electricity is of any use at all. And why did it not stop at 110 volts? That would be adequate to shock anything. Why such a super-electrician when none of the "higher" mammals ever "thought" of one?

The key question still remains: Where are all the thousands of intermediate bad-experiment electric eels? The other eels get along with no batteries at all, so all the ones with little or badly wired batteries must also be around—if they ever existed. But they do *not* exist. There are, in the waters of the earth, two or three electric fish, each a completely different design from the eel, each a member of a great family which has no batteries, and the intermediates do not exist. With no intermediates, how can there be evolution?

Another example is the poisonous snakes. They possess the most deadly armament in nature and to this day are still a menace. They provide an excellent example of FUNCTIONAL "Evolution." Non poisonous snakes are found all over the world as are poisonous snakes. They both survive perfectly and are supposed to be hundreds of millions of years old. But there are five times as many harmless as poisonous snakes. So here we have a very clear-cut case of two identical sub-families of the same species, one having a very fancy piece of self defense equipment which the other does not possess. That means natural selection could not operate. Now let's trace the details of this "evolution" which some ambitious poisonous snakes invented.

1. The idea of a poison injection system. No mammals, birds or fish and only one reptile have such a system. It is a luxury.

2. Develop a formula and a manufacturing process. The poison consists of some twelve very complicated and remote organic chemicals, which are designed exactly to match the nervous and circulatory systems of both cold-blooded and warm-blooded animals—at the same time. And a half drop can kill a man in an hour. They also have to be of exact viscosity, non-clogging, rapid diffusion, etc.

3. Design a plant to make the substance. A hundred Ph.D's, in a million dollar plant, might produce a shot with a thousand pounds of raw chemicals—if they knew how.

4. Build a piping system to pipe the poison, valves and all.

5. Build a very high pressure pump to pump it.

6. Design a tooth possessed by no other animal—in the shape of a hypodermic needle—and build a system to grow a new one speedily. (Why don't we "evolve" a third tooth? There have been billions of toothless persons. Why doesn't "nature" do something?)

7. Make connections to the circulatory and nervous systems; it must be timed to a tenth of a second.

But will this produce the poisonous species? Oh no! It must take all this material and incorporate it in the machinery that builds, in the egg, a machine that will enable the next snake to lay an egg that will produce the same thing. And a male and female snake must do all this together,

Furthermore, each snake is, as it must be, immune to his own poison, or die. How can it find the immunizing agent before it has the poison? But if it makes the poison first, it will drop dead and then be precluded from finding the agent!

There are some animals which, instead of fleeing like men and most animals from the deadly snakes, have the instinct built in them to attack and therefore, the snakes are subdued. Some of these animals are not immune to snake poison but survive because they know exactly how and where to bite. However, a few obscure animals are completely immune to snake poison. One is an obscure skunk and a few are non-poisonous snakes like the king-snake.

The implications of the foregoing are these:

1. The snake poison apparatus is an exceedingly complex chemical, mechanical, hydraulic, medical and engineering control device.

2. The snake has had no good reason to have evolved it.

3. An evolution requiring an animal to evolve within itself highly lethal substances is an impossibility.

4. The existence of just a few immune snake eaters, among animals bitten for millenia by snakes and still not immune, negates the "adaptation" ideology.

Of course, there is the magic word 'mutation.' That means that some ray comes by, and presto, the snake is transformed. Why? Because in the lab some insects exhibited minor changes when bombarded by X-rays. However, rays do not invent chemical formulae, piping systems or tooth-retracting mechanisms. But this is really very simple to dispose of; if any passing ray can so easily remodel the snake so drastically, there ought to be millions of vastly different species of snakes by now. There are not. And somehow, except for just that weapon and only a few minor differences, all snakes are very much alike. There are even poisonous and non-poisonous snakes which cannot be told apart.

Therefore, the poisonous snake could not have "evolved." And by all standards of logic we can prove that it did not. Because the millions of intermediate non-poisonous-to-poisonous snake species required to produce such an elaborate device do not exist. All poisonous snakes have the complete equipment. There ought to be at least a few degenerate species, having only remnants, but there aren't. Ergo-no evolution, no mutation, but Creation.

"Now how could so many scientists accept such a defective dogma? It has happened before that people made one-dollar theories with one-cent facts, and then, when fifty-cents worth of additional facts showed up, forgot to check again. Thus a false picture of nature has been built up. Given a few facts, the delusion called "evolution" is quickly blown away."

"If we now wake up from this false dream and truly comprehend that this world is the handiwork of the Creator, then, for the first time in history, we can begin to study and understand the mighty design of Creation. For only now do we have the scientific knowledge and

arduous disciplines that make it possible. From nature we can go to
the design of history and from there to man and his purpose and his
tasks. Though these are mighty problems, requiring great and dedi-
cated searching before the faint shadows of the design appear behind
the meaningless confusion of events, we also have the key, the Revelation, that alone can guide us through all errors."

The question that so-called scientists ignore is the perpetual heat and
light from the sun. My query is: Who is shoveling the coal to keep the sun
burning? Without the sun there can be no electric eels and no poisonous
snakes, and no life on earth. Who ignited the sun? Who determined that
93 million miles from earth was the correct distance to sustain life on
earth? Who keeps the concentration of oxygen in the atmosphere at exactly 21.5 per cent so that it never varies? Who created the first carbon
atom? When confronted by these questions the concept of evolution is
exploded as a fraud.

Dr. Morris Goldman, a parasitologist with the U.S. Public Health Service had this to say about evolution:*

"The dogma of evolution by natural selection of the most fit individuals is not a scientific theory because it is not susceptible to scientific testing. The theory that new species and entirely new kinds of
living creatures come into existence by random accumulation and
small variations has never been demonstrated scientifically either in
the laboratory or in the field . . . It is a doctrine resting on faith that
satisfies the secularist yearnings of our age."

The following was quoted from a chapter in A Science and Torah
Reader:**

"As far as Creation is concerned the true order of Creation does
not necessarily agree with the simple English translation of the Bible.
The Hebrew word "Yom" (day) used in the Biblical Creation account, is a day in G-d's eyes only, since man was not on earth, and
that a day in G-d's eyes might be a million years or more. In any
event, if the sky was created on the second "day" how are we to
understand what the first "day" consisted of in terms of time?"

"The Jewish calendar has as its beginning point 5730 years ago

---

starting *after* the week of Creation. So it is perfectly conceivable to say that the first seven days lasted billions of years, at least by man's yardstick of time. The actual length of the "six days of Creation" is immaterial since time is a relative and subjective concept. G-d created time and is therefore not subject to it. Until man was created at the end of the sixth day, time was passing only in the presence of G-d, and was therefore not subject to it. Until man was created at the end of the sixth day, time was passing only in the presence of G-d, and was therefore not observable or measurable for man."

"The Torah, the Five Books or Pentateuch was written by G-d. It is a book of moral laws, 613 of them, which tells man how to live a moral life in this world."

"The Torah speaks in the language of *contemporary* man, meaning regardless of which century or era, the language is comprehensible. It is written so that it has always been relevant and intelligible to every generation, from the former slaves in the Sinai desert four thousand years ago and to every generation since, up to and including the nuclear generation of today. At the same time, except for a specific number of rare instances, G-d's Torah has not revealed information which would overtly interfere with the historic evolution of mankind. Although the Torah describes the many instances in which G-d directly intervened in the unfolding of human history, they in no way interfered with man's ability to choose his own path. Human free will and freedom of action are fundamental concepts in the Jewish idea of man, as a being created in G-d's image."

"What does this tell us about the nature of the Torah and Jewish law? Essentially, the Torah expresses itself in the language which continues to be meaningful in each generation."

"Mankind has been delegated to explore and discover the world at his own pace. The raw materials of the universe were given to man to build with or destroy, as he chooses. The Divine Plan dictates that man unlock the secrets of the universe by effort and study. What the Torah did give man was the blueprint for the ideal type of *moral world* that he could build with these materials. If it had wished the Torah could have described Creation, for instance, in terms of nuclear physics; it could have described the "breath of life" in terms of biochemistry, but these descriptions would have been completely meaningless until the twentieth century, and would be completely incomprehensible to thirty centuries of humanity."

"Why didn't the Torah explain the ultimate truths of nuclear physics and biochemistry as part of the Creation story to make it understandable to each generation? Had it done so, the Torah would have interfered with and actually eliminated human progress. If the Torah had included the revelations of modern science, then they never would have been discovered by man. Had G-d revealed everything to the Jews on Sinai, the Jews would have immediately become the dominant nation in the world in the physical sense, instead of developing a moral sense. How could one attack with bow and arrows a nation that possesses the secrets of the atomic bomb? This superiority would also have forced the nations of the world to accept at least the truth and authenticity of the Torah because they would have no other logical way to explain what had happened. The course of history would have been radically altered, and man would have been denied his freedom of belief and action."

The second law of thermodynamics is entropy. This law states that anything left to itself tends to go from an orderly state to a disorderly state. For example, a motorcycle will become a heap of rust if left alone. A barn will disintegrate if not constantly repaired. Evolution contradicts this law. Evolution says that life, which is the highest form of *order* spontaneously arose from non-life or chaos, which is disorder. This is the reverse of entropy and makes a strong case for Creation. Evolutionists are trying desperately to fill the gaps (intermediate eels with only one battery) in the fossil record. If evolution is true there should be thousands of transition fossils like a half fish, a half amphibian, an eel with one battery instead of 500, but there are none.

To believe that a system as complex as the human digestive and reproductive systems could have developed on their own, without a guiding engineering intelligence (G-d) behind it, is another example of supreme human arrogance.

Let's examine the systems.

The creation of Adam and Eve as the progenitors of today's world population numbering in the billions, wherein one million new infants are born each day, requires two survival factors:

1. The presence of good teeth, and digestive system, to keep the *individual* alive. 2. The presence of a powerful, foolproof, reproductive system to keep the *race of mankind* alive.

The secret of how the digestive system converts food into energy that can be utilized by the body's muscles, has never been completely understood. It is still a mysteriously complex chemical, bacteriological process that has never been duplicated in the laboratory. The conversion of food into feces is a total mystery and has never been reproduced outside the human or animal intestine yet this complex process proceeds 24 hours a day without interference from voluntary control. The process is so miraculous that only a brilliant supernatural engineering, chemical, bacteriologist expert could design it. That expert can only be G-d. This had to be an infallible perfect system to assure the prolonged life of the individual, at least to the age of reproduction.

Now consider the reproductive system.

Both the male and female had to be designed to complete and fulfill each other with a drive as powerful as the hunger drive is to keep the individual alive.

Consider the vagina. Its walls are corrugated to provide the friction necessary to cause ejaculation in the male. It is lined with lubricating mucous cells to facilitate entrance of the penis. The entrance is sprinkled with Meissner's corpuscles, the function of which is to supply sensation of ecstatic pleasure when touched or stroked. These corpuscles were isolated in 1869 during an anatomical dissection by a German physiologist, named Georg Meissner, and occur nowhere else in the female body except around the vagina and nipples. Within the genetic code in the female body, the female develops a deep-seated longing and desire to have the vagina distended and filled by the male.

The fulfilling of the drive to have this blind tube called the vagina distended, has been instilled in the female brain at an anatomic point about which we know nothing. This compelling drive is in the genes of every female, and with it comes sensations called love, and develops within itself human addiction receptors. These receptors can be likened to the socket of a table lamp that requires an electric bulb to fulfill it. Once these receptors in the brain are filled up by the presence or the fellowship of the male, they become addicted to the male association. When the male suddenly breaks off the relationship either by death, or by an attraction to another female, the receptors which are no longer fulfilled, cause sensations of acute pain in the epigastric or upper abdomen and are, located specifically between the bifurcation of the ribs. A similar pain exists in morphine and heroin addicts when the drug is suddenly withdrawn from the patient. In the case of human addiction the existence of this unique pain which cannot be relieved by morphine, aspirin, or alcohol, serves an important reproductive purpose. The pain can only be relieved by the males reestablishing his relationship with the female which will ultimately lead to sexual intercourse with resultant propagation of the human race. This phenomenon is so powerful that it keeps psychiatrists busy making money in an attempt to alleviate the severe mental depression which accompanies this pain. The pain is not only associated with severe depression but also anorexia, loss of appetite, loss of ambition, and in some cases suicide.

The same phenomenon also occurs in the male who develops similar receptors for the female presence.

I have also sought truth in religion. The search for truth in this realm has occupied a long persistent search which involved extensive reading, detailed study of the major religions, including college courses in Christianity, Judaism, Islam, Buddhism, Zoroastrianism and Hinduism. I have attended seminars, listened to Yeshiva lectures, and spent weekends each summer for over 15 years enrolled in mountainside religious enclaves in Thurmont, Maryland. I have also read extensively in the philosophy of conservative, reform and orthodox Judaism.

After many years of deep thought and minute intellectual dissection I have concluded that I would not accept a religious belief based on the word of one man such as Joseph Smith who claimed he found some golden tablets which formed the basis of Mormonism or of Mary Baker Eddy and her concept of Christian Science.

Nor would I accept Christianity which was based on the word of Matthew, Mark, Luke and John who wrote of Jesus' life and events years after he died, all based on hearsay, and not eyewitnessed since Jesus himself never left any written records.

Buddhism, Hinduism and Zoroastrianism are a modern form of idol worship and represent a philosophy of life.

At some time in every individuals life the question of the creation of the universe and the origin of life, plagues man's mind. Why are we here, to what purpose, and why.

The stars and moon serve an exceedingly important service in the life of man. I once spent a night on the beach on a tiny, deserted island in the Caribbean near the island of Cozumel, Mexico. The island was uninhabited except for a family of raccoons. There was no artificial light, no electricity. There was no reflected light to the sky from a nearby city, and I was astounded to find that at midnight I could read the time on my watch by starlight. Later when the sky clouded up and obscured the stars I could still read my watch by the starlight which seemed to light up the clouds from behind. One does not often have an opportunity to observe this phenomenon in a city since light reflected from street lights on to clouds will prevent this observation even many miles from a city.

Without the stars the night would be as opaque as the total darkness in a photographic dark room, and neither man nor animals could take a single step without possible injury. Starlight, whether obstructed by clouds or not, provides sufficient light to guide man's steps safely on earth at night. The moon for much of the month provides additional light by reflecting light from the sun.

I was astonished to discover that the Creator of the moon also knew about the reflective properties of glass beads. We use tiny glass beads to coat the surface of movie screens, and to coat the white stripes that demarcate the center lines of our highways, and that coat the reflective STOP signs that our auto headlights light up at night. The astronauts who landed on the moon brought back buckets of the dust that covers the surface of the moon and analysts revealed the dust consisted of tiny glass beads!

Now who thought to cover the moon with glass beads?

Did this just happen by chance or was it planned?

In Antarctica there is an animal, the Emperor Penguin, that can only thrive in temperatures of 50° to 100° below zero. It stands on the ice for 38 days incubating an egg and its duck like feet never freeze. What prevents the Emperor Penguin's feet from freezing? In addition it must turn the newly laid egg which rests on top of its feet, every 12 minutes during these 38 days to maintain an even temperature so that the egg will properly incubate. The hot blood going to the Penguin's feet travels by arteries. The cold blood returning from the feet to the heart travels by veins, similar to the veins on the back of our hands. The specialized difference exists in the arteries. The arteries coil around the veins of the Emperor's feet and heat the cold blood returning to the heart. If this coiling did not exist the Penguin would freeze to death. This is known as counter-current heat flow and it exists mainly in the Emperor Penguin. The other 16 species of penguins which live in warmer climates do not possess this unusual system. Who designed this? Did it come about by itself or was there a Superior Intelligence which designed and placed into the genetic code of this particular penguin the ability to sustain life in temperatures so low that not even bacteria can survive. Even polar bears, which thrive in the warmer north polar regions, would perish in the coldest region on earth, the Antarctic.

These examples of brilliant planning are only a minuscule example inherent in the complex universe, none of which could have "just happened" all by itself. Nor could it have all come about by some mysterious explosion of gases in some far galaxy, a part of which cooled down to form the earth, from which appeared the Emperor Penguin, poisonous snakes and man himself.

The truth in religion for which I have searched and finally found is not at all complicated. It is detailed in the Books of Genesis, Exodus, Leviticus, Numbers, and Deuteronomy. In these books it relates that G-d, the Creator of the Universe is not man, does not think like man, and is totally different from any material or matter that exists in the entire Universe. This means that G-d does not, like man, consist of molecules or atoms or protons. That this Supreme Intelligence, known as G-d, is of a substance that does not exist anywhere in the Universe, and therefore man can never fathom what G-d is, because the human brain cannot visualize what does not and has never existed.

G-d created time, so He does not exist in a time frame and is not bound by time. G-d created the laws of gravity, of quantum mechanics, of atomic fission, of relativity so is not part of nor confined to any of these phenomenon.

This great, unknown Intelligent Force created man and his complex brain and endowed him with a free will. Adam, the first man had free will and misused it. The generation of man from Adam to Noah all had free will and misused it by living lives of lasciviousness, robbery, murder and adultery, lying and cheating.

G-d punished His creation in the flood and permitted Noah and his three sons to survive. The three races of mankind emerged from these three sons, Shem from whom came the white race, Japhet who gave rise to the yellow race, and Ham who was the progenitor of the black race of mankind.

How do we know this to be the truth? How do we know that G-d chose a particular people, the Hebrews, to become a nation that would tell the world of this phenomenon called G-d, and would teach the world how to channel man's free will into pathways of ethics, morality, and honesty?

For G-d to have created a universe and placed man in it without a set of rules or directions by which to live and not die by killing and robbing each other was as essential as providing oxygen in the atmosphere at exactly 21.5 per-cent.

For mankind to obey rules that curbed his free will, there had to be an event that made it unmistakably clear that it was G-d who demanded that man obey the rules, and not another man who made them up. For if rules of moral conduct which include the commandments not to commit robbery and adultery were drawn up by other men in one generation, what authority do these men have on subsequent generations? If man makes a rule involving morality and ethics, another man can change the rule since the authority is man. However, if G-d made the rule no man can change it.

This reasoning requires, of course, that G-d does exist, and that He alone gave the Ten Commandments besides the other 603 Commandments by which mankind was to live on this earth.

Judaism, the land of Israel, Jews, are all tied together for a special purpose, a mission. The Jews were selected by G-d not as a superior people, but simply to serve, to educate, to bring the message of the Commandments to humanity. The Jews were chosen by G-d to fulfill this mission. They were given the Land of Israel by G-d where they were to live the exemplary life as outlined in the 613 Commandments in the Torah, and by their example, the rest of mankind would learn the lessons of morality.

The Torah is the moral constitution of mankind.

The secular Jew who does not adhere to the Torah and its laws is theoretically without a mission. Today a majority of Jews know nothing of this mission, and worse still, the majority of Israeli Jews know nothing of this mission.

The Torah is not a book of fairy tales. The Torah made a contribution to the world that makes Einstein's Theory of Relativity pale into insignificance. The first major contribution it made consists of two words: God Exists. Prior to the Revelation at Mt. Sinai the world did not know this explosive fact. Both Islam and Christianity are derived from those two words.

The Torah revealed for the first time that man is created in G-d's image or form. This means man is not an animal and that he has free will; that man is independent of nature because of free will. Free will exists for man only, not for animals. Free will exists so man can choose the good since he has a choice to do good or evil. He cannot exercise this free ill in a vacuum or in space. So he must have form and an environment in which to exercise this free will, and both good and evil must exist in this environment. That's the way G-d created it together with a powerful commandment—"To choose good."

The Torah revealed that man is not just flesh and blood but that he has a soul, a spiritual self. This concept reflects the image of G-d.

The Torah for the first time in the history of mankind revealed the laws of morality. This cannot exist without the concept of G-d, without His higher authority to mete out punishment for failure to adhere.

The Torah revealed for the first time that mankind can speak to G-d through prayer, personally and without intermediaries. This had never before been heard in the entire world.

There has been no other work in the world to compare with this Torah. What the Bible or Torah did for mankind no other literature did for anyone in the world.

How do we know G-d gave these Commandments? If He appeared in some individual's dream state as Mohammed claims, then why believe Mohammed? He could have lied.

If G-d appeared to Moses in a burning bush or on a mountain top, why should we believe him? He could have been lying or deceived by his own imagination.

If G-d appeared to St. Paul and told him to spread the word of Christianity how do we know he wasn't lying?

If G-d appeared to Mary Baker Eddy, the founder of Christian Science or to Joseph Smith, the founder of Mormonism, how do we know they were not lying?

We do not know.

But G-d appeared to an assembly of over 600,000 Hebrews who *eyewitnessed* an event unheard of in history, and heard with their own ears, the Ten Commandments; who wandered for 40 years in the Sinai Desert, guided by a cloud by day and a mysterious overhead fire by night, and were fed manna for food, and provided with water, where it never existed and were told to do something so unbelievably impossible that if commanded to do this awful act by a man, would have instantly rebelled. Because this awful act was commanded by G-d, who they personally heard say it, it was done, and has been done without interruption to this day, because G-d commanded it which was eyewitnessed by half a million people and that event was not only dangerous, but painful. What was this awful command? Circumcision of all males.

When Paul was spreading the word of Christianity and doing his best to convince unbelievers, he was preaching a reform type of Judaism which was later called Christianity. The first thing he did was to throw out the commandment to circumcise all males. He made it easy to follow.

The important point here is that circumcision on the 8th day after birth was a Divine Commandment which has been performed among the Jews for over 3,000 years. This event of circumcision and the event of eating matzos or unleavened bread at the Passover Seder are events that have been observed continuously, since the commandment was given by G-d. The adherence to such a commandment in such a prolonged unbroken chain for over three millennia is unheard of in human history.

The Passover Seder is a religious occasion which fulfills two commandments: 1) to eat matzos to commemorate the exodus from Egypt and the escape from slavery to freedom; and the 2nd: to tell it (the story of the miracles associated with the Exodus from Egypt) to the children. The recounting of the exodus from Egypt, the 10 plagues and the parting of the Sea of Reeds has been told by father to son in an unbroken chain since the miraculous event occurred. Since it was eyewitnessed why should I not believe it. My father told it to me, his father to him, and so on through the generations all the way back to the actual event, also unheard of in human history. If the event of the Exodus was a fable and did not occur, could 500,000 of my ancestors have been fooled by a fast-talking Moses, who was tongue-tied by his own admission? And would they have accepted the barbaric unheard of command to circumcise all males when even today, hemorrhage is a grave complication of this operation? Before the Israelites entered the promised land, all adults had to be circumcised. And today we have recently been shown that on the 8th day the blood clotting mechanisms become manifest, not on the 6th or 7th, but on the 8th day.

Three thousand years ago circumcision was unheard of. There was no previous experience with this operation to even ascertain that circumcision on the 8th day would be safer since doing the operation before the 8th day would lead to uncontrolled hemorrhage and death. In hospitals today non-Jewish parents who desire circumcision for their infants for health reasons frequently leave the hospital on the 4th or 5th day. If they want the child circumcised before he leaves the hospital with the mother, it is now necessary to inject the child with a blood clotting chemical known as Vitamin K, to keep him from hemorrhaging, despite careful tying off of all the bleeding vessels at the time of surgery.

Naturally, the Creator of the universe and of the blood-clotting mechanisms, commanded the 8th day for circumcision.

Since circumcision was an unknown entity over 3,000 years ago how else would one explain this Commandment, one of the 613? And so specific is this commandment that even if the 8th day falls on the Sabbath or Yom Kippur, the operation must be performed on that day.

This law has been observed since the time of Moses when it was commanded at Mt. Sinai, in an unbroken chain, and never has there been a lapse in its observance through all these centuries. If such a law was commanded by man would we today even think of doing such an unwarranted surgical procedure on our new-born babies? To the Jew, circumcision is not a health commandment, it is a directive from G-d himself which was commanded as the signing of a contract between G-d and the Jewish people for all generations until eternity.

Non Jews are not obligated to be circumcised. If this were a Commandment to preserve the health of a child, G-d would have created man without a prepuce since man was created as a perfect creature.

Why does so much of the world's college-educated population refuse to admit that a force superior to man exists in the universe? Resistance to the concept of G-d as the Creator of all that exists in the world including the sun and stars and planets, including all of physics, chemistry, and mathematics in addition to all the moral and ethical laws, stems from man's arrogance. It is a challenge to man's pretensions to self-sufficiency and to all the strategies that he has devised to sustain them. Man cannot deal with any force superior to himself. If he accepts this force he takes on a serious responsibility. He must not lie, steal, cheat or commit adultery. If he does, punishment is sure to follow. That is what the Creator of the Universe told this multitude of 500,000 people. Life is so much simpler without G-d looking over one's shoulder.

The eyewitnessed event that happened before the eyes of half a million people who had been enslaved in Egypt cannot be lightly dismissed. These people saw and heard the essence of the Creator of the Universe. They witnessed an event in which G-d spoke directly to them. The difficulty in man's acceptance of this unusual event is that man today did not experience it, and Bible critics report this event as the imaginings of ancient historians. The essential difference between reform and orthodox Judaism concerns this event. Reform Jews do not believe this occurred. Orthodox Jews believe it did occur. If it did not occur then the entire Jewish Orthodox Religion is a myth and a fraud, as is Christianity and Islam which are based on this event.

Did G-d appear to this multitude of slaves just released from Egypt?

The following are my beliefs as to why this is a true event:

1. I accept the fact that a Superior Force, unlike anything in the universe, exists. This force is called G-d. And that this force who created the universe, and man, actually appeared at Mt. Sinai to give to mankind a moral law to guide his conduct on this earth so that men would not kill each other.
2. Since G-d is not of atoms, or molecules, we can never know the secret of His essence.
3. We can accept the fact of man as creator of beautiful things such as Tiffany glass, sculptures and paintings by Michel Angelo and beautiful buildings such as the Taj Mahal in India, but when it comes to man's brain, the supreme achievement of creation, non-

believers claim this came about by itself; it evolved; that no creator was necessary. This is the supreme example of man's arrogance and I cannot accept such an arrogant and egocentric belief.

4. Since I accept that G-d created the universe and all the natural laws including time, I can, therefore, with facility, accept that G-d can alter his creation as an architect can alter his blueprint, or a builder his building, as He sees fit.

5. It was, therefore, no great feat for G-d to have parted the Reed Sea when the Israelites departed Egypt. This event was also eyewitnessed by a half million people.

6. It was no great feat for G-d to have led the Israelites through the Sinai Desert, guided by an overhead fire by night, a cloud by day, and the provision of manna to feed this multitude for 40 years. I have been in the Desert of Sinai and it is as barren as the Sahara. The clothes and shoes of those who left Egypt never wore out. The entire event was a miracle. A miracle is an event outside of the natural law of which man is aware. It is, therefore, logical that if G-d created the laws of gravity, of atomic fission, of quantum mechanics, He can alter them at will. G-d altered the laws of nature during the ten plagues that tested Pharoah. He altered the laws of nature when Joshua crossed the Jordan on dry land to occupy the land of Canaan which is today the State of Israel. All of these miracles are possible and quite simple for the Creator of the Universe to perform. Two examples of a modern-day miracle is the 1948 Israeli War of Independence when the entire Arab world was defeated by a tiny group of people who were not even galvanized into a nation. And the Six-Day War in 1967 when every military expert in the world predicted the downfall of Israel because of the superior power of seven Arab nations sworn to drive every Israeli into the Mediterranean Sea. What happened could only be the result of divine intervention. Israel defeated the Arab nations and would have conquered all of Egypt and Syria if the United States and the USSR had not called a halt. When the Prime Minister, Golda Meir, was questioned about the victory, instead of attributing it to a divine miracle she merely said, "Our soldiers are well-trained." But Golda Meir was not a believer in G-d, nor was she an orthodox Jew.

7. The vastness of the Universe, the infinity of space, is a testament to G-d's all-encompassing power, and to man's puny finiteness.

8. The Bible is not propaganda. Egyptian hieroglyphics did not mention the Exodus from Egypt because ancient nations recorded only their successes, never their failures.

9. Millions of people today believe in the Biblical miracles such as the 10 plagues, the miracle of Manna, the division of the Sea of Reeds, and the Revelation at Sinai. This belief is based on a chain of believers in these events. How did this chain get started? The truth of this is based on the psychological principle that if a possible event really occurred it would have left behind enormous, easily available evidence of its occurrence. If the evidence did not exist, people would not believe it since there is a limit to gullible belief. A public miracle cannot start in the absence of social evidence such as an eyewitness report. People will not believe this unless it happened to all of their ancestors. This eyewitnessed happening is made compelling by calmness, repetition, corroboration, irrelevance of expertise and absence of self interest.

The miracle of Manna, for example, which fell each day for 39 years after the Exodus from Egypt fulfilled all of the above criteria, calmness, corroboration, repetition, etc.

10. Regarding the Revelation by G-d at Sinai, no other religion in the world claims that G-d revealed himself and spoke to an entire nation who eyewitnessed the event. If there is no public theophany there has to be a private holy man, or an inspired man, and this is *not* evidence. This individual could be lying or hallucinating. If the evidence does not exist people will not believe it. It was never a goal in Judaism to accept the truth of Judaism on faith. It is based on *eyewitnessed evidence*. Christianity and Islam teach a distrust of reason and evidence and base their religious belief solely on faith.

The Torah, or the five books of Moses, is known as the written law. It contains, besides the Ten Commandments, 603 additional Commandments which Jews are obligated to observe. This Torah, like the Constitution of the United States, was written for all generations, from the time of Moses unto eternity. At the time the Torah was given by G-d to Moses and the Israelites, an oral law was also given by G-d to Moses who taught it to Aaron, the heads of the tribes, and to Joshua who became the leader at the death of Moses. This Oral law was written down in the second century C.E. and was known as the *Mishna*.

Non-Jews are under no obligation to observe these laws. However, there were seven laws which, according to the oral tradition, were given to Adam, and have become known as the Seven Noachide Laws which all mankind was obligated to observe. These laws are as follows:

1. Not to murder
2. Not to commit adultery
3. Not to worship idols
4. Not to steal or rob
5. Not to eat a limb or flesh torn off a live animal
6. To appoint judges in each generation.
7. Not to curse G-d.

A non-Jew who observes these seven laws is considered by G-d to be as excellent an individual as the Jew who observes all 613 laws (which includes these Seven Noahidic Laws).

It is for this reason that a non-Jew who desires to convert to Judaism is discouraged from doing so by Orthodox Rabbis. He must point out to the candidate for conversion that it is unnecessary to assume the burden of 613 commandments when all one has to observe is the Seven Noachide Laws. A convert must refrain from working on the Sabbath; must not eat crabs, shrimp, lobster, pork and meat from any animal unless it has a cloven hoof and chews the cud, must fast on Yom Kippur; eat only unleavened bread during the eight days of Passover; must not sleep in the same bed with his wife during her menstrual period and for seven days after that, and if a male wishes to convert he must go through a painful operation—circumcision.

Unlike other religions, Judaism today does not seek converts. In early Rabbinic times, however, Judaism was a missionary religion. Later it stopped seeking converts because the church prohibited it.

During recent centuries, men of science have given much time to studying the works of creation. What have they concluded? One of the pioneers in the field of electricity, the well-known British physicist Lord Kelvin, declared: "I believe the more thoroughly science is studied the further does it take us from anything compared to atheism." The European-born scientist Albert Einstein, though reputed to an an atheist, confessed: "It is enough for me to . . . reflect upon the marvelous structure of the universe, which we can dimly perceive, and to try humbly to comprehend even an infinitesimal part of the intelligence manifest in nature." The American scientist and Nobel prize winner Arthur Holly Compton said: "An orderly unfolding universe testifies to the truth of the most majestic statement ever uttered—'In the beginning God.' He was quoting the opening words of the Bible.

CHAPTER V

ISRAEL AND THE ARABS

In 1987 I decided to lend a helping anesthesia hand to the State of Israel since it is the land of my ancestors. As it was a struggling new nation, I thought I should contribute whatever talent I possessed.

On a previous visit in 1986, the Minister of Health assured me that my services would be more than welcome since I would not require the state to pay me. I offered to work as a volunteer. I had visited several dental clinics and those in charge were most enthusiastic about my returning in 1987 to place under conscious sedation those unmanageable children who otherwise would be untreatable.

I obtained a leave of absence from Johns Hopkins, and approximately nine months before going to Israel I made application through the Ministry of Health for a permit to do this work. I was assured that by the time I arrived in Israel all the red tape and bureaucratic preparations would be completed, a work permit would be ready, and to work I would go.

This did not happen. I ran into other non-Israeli physicians and psychologists who have been waiting literally for years and their permits are still pending.

This impenetrable brick wall of bureaucracy existing in Israel is so ridiculous, time consuming, frustrating, and impossible to comprehend, that those caught in its net can only shake their heads in disbelief. There were forms in triplicate, forms in duplicate, forms in quadruplicate, each requiring a passport-size photo. I spent days standing in line A, only to discover I should have been in line A of an adjoining building, and usually in a building on the other side of town. To attempt to obtain information via telephone as to the correct building, which floor and which line to stand in, is impossible since the voice at the other end of the line speaks only Hebrew, when one can get the line. The busy signal is as predictable as the beautiful bluest blue sky that hovers over Jerusalem in summer. To get to the other building involves trying to find a cab, or if in one's own rented car, one is faced with bumper to bumper traffic without a place to park. This is especially pleasant when you find yourself inhaling the exhaust of an old Egged Bus, in a traffic line two blocks long with no opportunity of maneuvering out of the line, since the streets in Jerusalem are narrow.

In a state of partial Egged asphyxiation one arrives at the "other" building and stands in line. There's always a line. My turn comes. The harassed, bureaucratic clerk says everything is in order, but "I'll need your birth certificate." "No one told me that was required," I say. The clerk does not comprehend English. Someone in line translates the drama into Hebrew for the clerk and his answer into English for me.

In high dudgeon I leave the building and complain to the Minister of Health via phone about the impossibility of coping with such disorganized bureaucracy. He assures me he will do what he can and to please have patience.

Meanwhile weeks go by and nothing seems to be happening. The irony of the situation is that I was asked to come to Israel to introduce concepts that we were employing at Johns Hopkins, and I agreed to do this gratis.

While waiting for my permit to hurdle the bureaucratic brick wall I decided to apply for a driver's license.

Applying for an Israeli driver's license is a typical case history of bureaucratic adventure into frustration, anger, hopelessness and cephalalgia.

Any normal person would phone the licensing bureau to determine hours, procedures, and the necessary documents to have at hand. In Israel this is impossible. The phone is always busy, apparently there is only one trunk line. This necessitates a personal visit to the motor vehicle bureau in Jerusalem located in a section known as the industrial zone.

After impossible traffic I pass the railroad station, head out to the Bethlehem Road, and after many stops for directions I find the bureau. I park. I enter the building, a one-story, Jerusalem-stone building where bedlam reigns supreme.

Everyone is yelling, there are six lines of sweating Arabs, rabbis, pregnant women, trying to restrain their two year olds, representatives of every country in the world—blond Norwegians, black Sephardim, Chinese, disgusted-looking New Yorkers, and young hippies in short shorts and shorter tops.

I begin asking the last person in each line where do I apply for a driver's license. No one speaks English. I try Yiddish. Someone responds. Go to line Gimmel.

Twelve people are ahead of me in line Gimmel, all dripping sweat in this non-air-conditioned furnace in the month of July. Not being British I can't tolerate queues. I wiggle my way to the head of the line and ask the clerk in English if this is the correct line for applying. Without looking up she answers sluggishly, since she is also suffering from the heat, "ken" which means "yes" in Hebrew. To the back of the line I now stand. I wait. And wait. And wait. Soon there is loud shouting at the head of the line. The clerk has disappeared, ten minutes have elapsed, and she has not returned. No one chances to leave his place in line since she may return any second. Three lines away another female clerk disappears and that line starts to scream and bellow. Two other clerks leave from other lines to try to find the original two departees. Soon four lines of 12 people are all screaming, waving their arms and complaining about the lousy service and asserting that the clerks do not care about their neighbors; yet, no one dares leave his place in line. Soon the harassed clerks return, probably from drinking a coke in their recreation room, and the bedlam subsides. There is never less than 12 in the line that extends to the wall so that no one else can squeeze in.

An hour later I reach the clerk. I show her my Maryland driver's license and tell her I would like an Israeli license. "But you are in the wrong line," she says, "You must go to line Aleph for an application." "But you yourself told me this was the right line. Can't you hand me an application so I do not have to go to the end of line Aleph?" I say. "It's impossible," she says. And I tell her, "I'm drenched in sweat."

So for another hour I stand in line Aleph and resolve that I will communicate this inefficiency to the Director of Motor Vehicles.

After much discussion with other frustrated individuals I discover that these clerks cannot be fired, that the unions control job security, and that complaints fall on deaf ears. This is the British system that was set up from early socialist days and further complicated by Ben-Gurion-type bureaucracy from Poland, Russia and Roumania, and that's the way it will remain.

My turn comes. I receive the application. The clerk says you must go to optometrist for an eye examination. But I had one in the United States and you have it in your files, I respond. It must be done here. In which line do I go after the eye exam? Right here in this line. Are you certain that's all I need, no other documents? That is all she says.

I leave the building in a state of acute dehydration determined to somehow beat this bureaucracy.

The next day for $2.50 I receive a cursory eye examination by an optometrist from South Africa. He fills out the form for me.

Once again, I proceed through the impossible traffic and suffering from asphyxiation from Egged bus exhaust, I arrive at the motor vehicle bu-

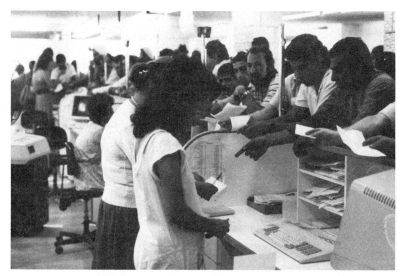

Lines of irate applicants for driver's licenses at the Bureau of Motor Vehicles in Jerusalem.

reau. I enter the building. There is bedlam again. The six lines are eternal. I take my place against the wall of line Aleph and wait and sweat, and wait.

An hour later I reach the same clerk behind the glassed-in counter. Here is my Maryland license and my official eye exam.

What she told me I could not believe. "Our computers just went down and you'll have to return tomorrow." I felt like screaming and bellowing like all the other Israelis. But I didn't. With a feeling of hopeless frustration I once again left that awful building.

The next day I went immediately to the head of the line to determine that the computers were "up." They were. Back to the wall, the sweat, the heat, the noise, children screaming, other lines arguing with clerks.

Finally I meet my friendly clerk. "Boker tov" she greets me in Hebrew. She looks over my application. Everything is in order, she says, but since you are over 60 you will need a physical examination. But I had one in the U.S. and you have that. It must be by an Israeli physician. Why didn't you tell me this four lines and four days ago. That's the way it is she says. Are you sure you do not want me to bring my Bar Mitzvah certificate, my divorce papers, a statement from a psychiatrist saying I'm normal. Please tell me so the next line will be the last line.

I consider using taxis rather than driving my own car. I consider flying back to the U.S. and never returning here again. Maybe another week end in Eilat will calm me down.

The wait in a physician's office was almost as bad as the lines at the motor bureau.

Fortunately on the final day at the motor bureau I had to endure only one 12-line wait. The cute clerk said you haven't given up, have you? We will mail your license to you. Shalom. And so ended the ordeal of obtaining a driver's license.

Applying for a telephone, protesting an incorrect tax bill or any activity involving the Government of Israel requires standing in line, sweating, waiting and multiple returns to the same office until the business is completed. That's how bureaucracy in Israel operates.

There is only one bureaucracy that is not only efficient, but is superefficient. That's the police department.

I rented a Hertz car in Jerusalem and being unable to read the parking and no parking signs, I parked my car wherever I could. Parking space simply does not exist since the city of Jerusalem was not planned for automobiles.

A car parked in a no parking zone will, it seems, within minutes, get the iron boot known as a "wheel-lock". To get it removed one has to walk or take a taxi to the Seon Co., Ltd. at 12 Shammai Street in Jerusalem. They will unlock the boot for a fee, usually 26 sheckels or $15.60. After paying the fee you must return to your auto and wait for the key man who unlocks it.

Since the key man was just leaving the building with a stack of 12 paid orders to unlock boots, I asked if he could drive me to my car. Sure he said, follow me. When we arrived at his small truck he had a summons on his windshield for illegal parking, but no iron boot since he had them all. I told him I did not mind paying the fee since the fine helps the State of Israel.

So as not to waste my time I enrolled in the Ohr Somayach Tanenbaum College in Jerusalem which features a summer program in philosophy and religion. Lectures are given daily by outstanding scholars.

To my surprise one of the lectures was a professor of philosophy from Johns Hopkins, Dr. David Gottlieb who now makes Jerusalem his home.

Aside from the impossible bureaucracy which has infected every aspect of life in Israel from applying for a telephone to getting an automobile inspected, there are enormous positive aspects to living in Israel.

It takes 20 minutes to drive from the traffic snarl which is Jerusalem, to the peacefulness, loneliness, unspeakable beauty of the barren solitude which is the road to the Dead Sea, the lowest point on earth, being 285 feet below sea level, and totally surrounded by high, barren, rock mountains.

To reach the Dead Sea one traverses undulating, rock-strewn hills where reside Beduins in their black, goat-hair tents, stray camels, and herds of goats. Within 10 minutes one is in a fairy land so remote from Jerusalem that it is difficult to believe that suddenly, as if transfixed, you are in this vast lonely desert, where no one can live except the Beduin because of the heat. The pathways, the surroundings are the same as they were in the Biblical times of Joshua. And you realize this as the inexorable heat of the sun bakes the earth, the air and the interior of your automobile. Soon the road sign points to Jericho, the oldest city in the world. Further on is the Dead Sea, glistening in its deep purple grandeur. On the Arab side of the sea are the mountains of Moab and the highest peak is probably Mt. Nebo where no man has ever found the spot where G-d buried Moses.

You soon come to realize that this little country known as Israel has so many attributes that the traffic, exhaust fumes of its cities and the impossible bureaucracy are miniscule compared to the natural resources of this land.

There are canyons as deep as the Grand Canyon in Mitzpah Ramon; there are four seas, the Mediterranean, the Red Sea at Eilat, and the Dead Sea and the Sea of Galilee. There are snow-capped peaks at Mt. Hermon in the North, and a man-made mountain in the midst of the desert built by Herod 2,000 years ago known as Herodion. The top of this high peak, the highest in the vicinity of Jerusalem, was recently excavated and found to be a haven of refuge for King Herod who built the mountain from the desert floor up, and on its top a synagogue was found plus a mikva, sauna baths and much more. I climbed to the top of this mountain in July and the view of the spires of Jerusalem to the north and the Dead Sea to the east was one of the most spectacular sights I have ever seen. Another one of King Herod's hiding out spots was Masada where excavations revealed similarities to Herodion.

I went to Eilat, a new city located at the extreme north end of the Red Sea. The Red Sea at this point is like an inverted ∩. This ∩ is divided right down the center. On the west side is Eilat, and the mountains of the Sinai desert where the Israelis wandered for 40 years. On the right side

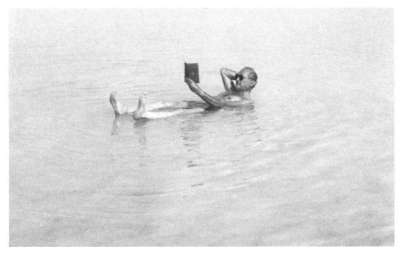

Reading a book while floating in the Dead Sea. The salts in the water are so supersaturated that it's impossible to sink. Arthritis sufferers find relief because of the high concentration of bromide salts which are absorbed and act as an analgesic.

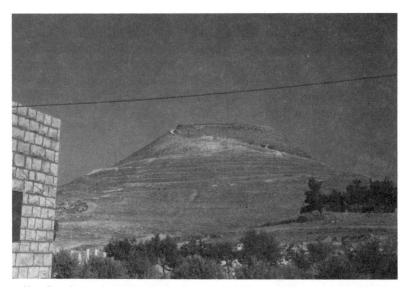

Herodian. A manmade mountain constructed from the desert floor up by King Herod in the First Century B.C.E. as a fortress to protect himself from attack. Masada was another of his escape points of refuge.

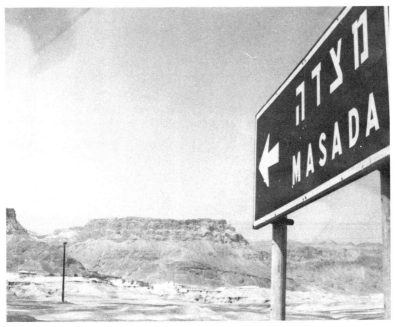

Masada, another of King Herod's mountain top escape aeries.

across the mid line is Aqaba, a Jordanian enemy city just waiting to pounce on this west bank and gobble up the real estate, the hotels, the desalination plants, the condominiums, and the oil-receiving docks. The mountains on the Arab side are the mountains of Saudi Arabia which follow the sea until it expands into the Arabian Sea a hundred miles to the South.

Israel won the entire Sinai desert in the six-day war of 1967. After winning a decisive victory over an aggressive enemy, Egypt plus Syria and Jordan, Israel did something that no nation in history has ever done. It gave the Sinai Desert with its vast oil reserves, plus Mt. Sinai where the Torah was given by G-d to the Israelites, back to Egypt. The prime minister of Israel at that time was Menachim Begin. The President of Egypt was Anwar Sadat. Now Sadat is dead and the peace between Egypt and Israel is precarious at best, since a new president in an Arab country appears not to be bound by the word of a former, dead president.

There is a city to the south of Jerusalem known as Hebron. It is a city that has been continuously viable for over 2,000 years. Today it is occupied by Arabs, over 60,000 of them, and they surround a tiny enclave of

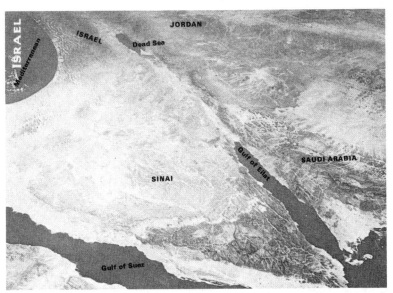

View from a satellite showing the relationship between Israel, Jordon, Sinai, and Saudi Arabia.

40 Jewish families who are orthodox, and devoted to the cause that Jews should live in Israel wherever they are needed. The importance of Hebron to the Jew is a building whose stone walls are over 2,000 years old, the huge blocks of which were laid at the same time as the Temple Wall in Jerusalem during the reign of King Solomon. This building has been preserved through century after century because it was a building containing something holy to both Jews and Moslems. It contains the graves of Abraham, Isaac, and Jacob, the forefathers of the entire Jewish people, and their wives Sarah, Leah, and Rebekah. The Arabs also venerate Abraham since he is also the forefather of the Arabs. The Biblical story details how Abraham married a second wife, Hager, a handmaiden of his first wife Sarah, because Sarah was barren. Hagar became pregnant with Ishmael and Sarah had her sent away. Ishmael was the first Arab and from him came all the other Arabs. Sarah later bore a child in her later years, Isaac, and this marked the origin of the Jewish people. Abraham was thus the first Jew, and the father of the Arab people as well.

This building known as the Cave of Machpelah resembles a medieval church. The major portion of the inside is simply open space covered by large rugs where the Arabs pray to Allah by kneeling and prostrating themselves on the rugs.

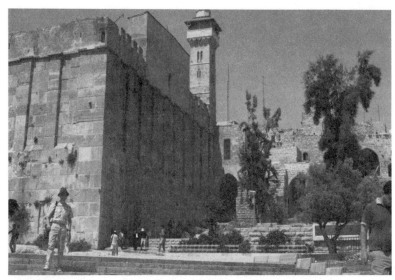

The "Cave" of Machpelah in Hebron. Abraham, Isaac and Jacob the forefathers of the Jewish People are buried below this structure, the walls of which are as old as the Wailing Wall in Jerusalem.

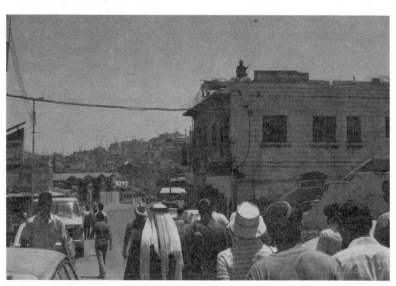

Hebron, where Arabs are in the majority, where only 40 Jewish families reside, where Israeli soldiers patrol the city even from roof tops with Uzzi guns.

It was not until 1967, after the Six-day War, that the Jews could enter this so-called cave. For hundreds of years prior to 1967, the Jew could only ascend the first seven steps of the entrance and there say his prayers, whereas the Arab had access to the entire structure.

Since 1967 a portion of the inside now houses a small synagogue where Jews come to pray.

What confuses me is this: The Israelis won the war, and instead of limiting the Arabs to only seven steps, they permitted the Arabs to control the entire structure and only a very tiny room was allotted to Jews as a synagogue. It portends giving the Sinai back to Egypt after Israel won the Sinai in the war.

Glancing up to the top of surrounding building one sees a sight quite menacing to the Arabs. Israeli soldiers with high-powered rifles guard the entire area around the Cave of Machpelah. Not only from the roofs of apartment houses but on the ground, Israeli soldiers with Uzzi guns are on constant duty. I spoke to one of the soldiers and asked him if he harbored fears of being knifed in the back, a favorite behavior of his Arab cousins. He said, "If one of us is killed here in Hebron, the Arabs just know there would be a wholesale massacre of every Arab in sight. No, we're not afraid of them. They're afraid of us."

Israel is a country where almost every fruit and vegetable known to mankind grows somewhere within its seven climatic zones. It has every variety of scenery, every variety of kosher edible fish, it now manufactures almost every item it needs for building houses, including plastics, glass, hardware, roofing, toilets, bathtubs, furniture, rugs, towels, blankets, space heaters and a hundred other items. Israel is now manufacturing its own military aircraft, guns (Israel has one of the world's best guns and exports them) bullets, and the Arabs know Israel may have the atomic bomb and the know-how to deliver it. All that from a dried-out-desert, rock-strewn country within a space of 40 years. And with all of the impeding bureaucracy one wonders how was this ever accomplished?

But its political-religious system is a lesson in social schizophrenia.

Jewish leaders throughout the world are chosen not for their piety, nor for their knowledge of Judaism, but for their ability to raise money.

Jews enjoy attacking the Christian world, the Vatican, Roosevelt, and Churchill for not helping the Jews during the Nazi Holocaust. Since 1976, 80,000 Christians have been murdered in Lebanon and what did the Christian world do for Christians? Nothing. And why should we expect the Christian world to help Jews. The real tragedy is not what Christians did not do for Jews, the tragedy is what Jewish leaders did not do for

Jews. In 1942, three years before the Holocaust ended, while four million Jews were still alive, American Jewish leaders like Stephen Wise knew that 12,000 Jews each day were being gassed to death. It is no secret that Jews in Germany pleaded with American Jews to influence Roosevelt to bomb the railroad lines and bridges leading to the death camps. This would delay the cattle cars full of Jews by 12,000 each day.

In 1986, dozens of Jews were arrested outside the White House in Washington protesting apartheid in Africa. Did one Jew chain himself to the White House fence protesting the death of 12,000 Jews each day in Germany?

Stephen Wise, knowing details of the tragedy chose to remain silent. He said Roosevelt told him to be silent so as not to make this a Jewish war, that would cause anti-Semitism. That's why Jewish leaders were silent in the 1940's. They were afraid of anti-Semitism! They were afraid of what the gentiles would say. For that they remained silent while 12,000 of their fellow Jews were dying each day. In 1948, I was in Auschwitz and saw with my own eyes the tons of hair clipped from the heads of women prior to their going to the gas chamber, to be used in pillows and mattresses, in addition to all the other horror scenes that were preserved at the time, only three years after the war was ended.

The State of Israel has a real problem, a problem of schizophrenia, because it is attempting to build a Zionist state and a democratic state and the two are incompatible.

What is Zionism? Zionism is the movement to create a Jewish state. A Jewish state means a state with a majority of Jews, where Jews are in the majority and in control of their destiny.

The Declaration of Independence of the State of Israel is one of the most famous schizophrenic documents of all times. The moving paragraph of that document states the following: "We hereby proclaim the establishment of a Jewish State." Two paragraphs later it says: "Equal political rights for all inhabitants regardless of nationality or religion." This is a clear contradiction of the first paragraph.

The problem is, do the Arabs have the right to sit quietly and start throwing stones at buses not to speak of grenades and bombs in Israeli supermarkets. Do they have a right to be a majority in Israel? Of course they do. This is democracy according to the second paragraph in the constitution.

There is an enormous contradiction here. You cannot have a Zionist State, a Jewish State and call it a democracy. This is an impossibility. The Arab birthrate is four times that of the Jews. The Arabs have babies and the Jews have abortions. Arabs don't have abortions because they're religious! Today emigration from the United States has dried up. The Jews are leaving Israel in droves. The Galilee already has a majority of Arabs who hate the Jews. Cities like Ramalla, Nablus, Acco, and Jaffa all have Arab majorities. Today there are seven Arabs in the Knesset who speak Hebrew like everyone else, who are *sabras* and skilled and arrogant. The worst part of the problem is that the secular Jewish liberals have such concern for Arabs that all we have to do, they say, is raise the Arab living standards and then they'll be *good* Arabs. The liberals proclaim that the Arabs have more indoor toilets than any Arabs in the Middle East. Is there one Arab in Israel who will let his national pride be sold for a thousand toilets? Does the Arab care that he has indoor plumbing?

In 1955, a law of return was passed in Israel. It says, any Jew has an automatic right to come to Israel. Could a law such as this be passed today in Israel's democratic Knesset? It would be condemned as racist. Is there one Israeli Arab who enjoys singing his national anthem, which is Hatikva, which translates into "The Soul of a Jew Yearns."

The constant repetition of the U.J.A. (United Jewish Appeal) liberal speakers tell how the Jews came here and transformed a desiccated desert into a garden. The Arab says it was my desert, now it's your garden.

The Arabs want to do away with Israel. That is the most important fact of life that I realized during my sojourn in this schizophrenic country.

There is a "Peace Now" movement here in Israel, the object of which is to give back to the Arabs the West Bank, and the Gaza District. They think this will buy peace as Menachim Begin thought when he gave the Sinai back to Egypt.

When they had the West Bank in the 1920's the Arabs rioted. Why did they murder 67 Jews in one day in 1929? Between 1936 and 1938, 510 Jews were massacred in Israel. In 1947 they turned down the partition plan passed by the United Nations, went to war and killed 6,000 Jews when they already had the West Bank.

King Hussein of Jordan is a moderate Arab seeking peace! He makes it clear each day that he will not sign any peach treaty unless Israel gives up all the territory of the West Bank including East Jerusalem. Then there will be peace, he says. The question is who had the West Bank and East Jerusalem in 1967 before the Six Day War? The Hadassah?

Hussein had it and he went to war. Is this logical? Or is it because he wanted West Haifa, and West Tel Aviv and all the real estate west to the Mediterranean. Why? He fought because he thought he could win. That's what Hussein wants now.

What is the answer to this problem which will never go away unless remedial action is taken now before the Arab population explosion votes Israel out of existence. Then, through the vote and the democratic process that our liberal secular leaders praise so highly, they vote themselves a Palestinian State wherein the Jews have no say whatsoever.

The answer to this burning question puzzles me and opinions vary as to what action to take. The Kach party in Israel has one answer. The other parties have not yet stopped arguing among themselves. Here is what the Kach party advocates:

1. The Arabs can remain in Israel but as non-citizens. They will have personal rights, religious rights, social rights—but no national rights. They will not serve in the Knesset, in the army or in the government. They will have nothing to say about running the country. If they agree to this they can stay.

2. Those who do not agree with this will have to leave quickly and quietly and will be compensated for their property.

3. Those who refuse to go will be put on trucks and transported right across the Jordan, right into King Hussein's back yard.

Is this an acceptable modern method of dealing with an unwanted, dangerous population. The Kach Party points out that a similar exchange of population occurred in 1947 between India and Pakistan. And in 1945, 13 million Germans were thrown out of Czechoslovakia and Poland— Germans who had lived there for over 1,000 years. The Poles and Czechs had enough of that master race.

What immediate result would occur? Jews will not be murdered each week, and fear will not stalk the buses, and markets, and streets and highways of the Jewish State. And the overpopulation of Arab babies will no longer threaten the very existence of the Jewish State.

If the Arabs become a majority what will happen to American Jewish investment in Israel such as the hotels, real estate, chemical factories, yeshivas, and the Israeli Army itself. And who will prevent the Arabs from changing the name from Israel, a Jewish state, to Palestine, an Arab state?

What will the world say about this? That's not the question. The question is what will America say? America can't say a word since America usually supports dictators such as Franco in Spain and Salazar in Portugal. Countries don't back countries because of friendship. They do so for national interest only. America's interest in Israel is the Haifa Naval base.

The Negev is filled with U.S. arms in case of War with the USSR. America's interest in Israel is access to the oil of the Middle East. America will cry crocodile tears to assuage the Arabs for about two days until another "gate" occupies the headlines. What other choice does America have in this region besides Israel? Kuwait? Oman? Saudi Arabia? Aba Dabi? Jordan?

In Jerusalem today there are over 140,000 Arabs. Romli has 33% Arabs, Lydda has 25% Arabs. Hebron is almost 100% Arabs. Israeli Jews who are brain washed by the Palestine (Jerusalem) Post think they can wish this problem away. From 110,000 Arabs in 1948, there are 730,000 in Israel today. Arab babies are subsidized through the National Health Insurance system which pays every Arab mother for every baby she has.

The essence of the struggle in Israel is not between the Jew and the Arab, it is between the secular or non-religious Jew and his conscience. He awakens each day ridden with guilt that he is a thief, that he stole Israel from the Arabs. This secular Jew, who incidentally forms the majority of Israel's population, desperately attempts to sooth his aching conscience by supporting the Arabs on every possible issue.

Some definitions are in order to define the difference between a religious Jew, a secular Jew, an ultraorthodox Jew and a reform, conservative or reconstructionist Jew.

A man or woman born of a Jewish mother is always a Jew, regardless of affiliation. The word Jew denotes a religion, not a culture and not national state affiliation such as French, Spanish or Japanese.

A religious or orthodox Jew believes in G-d, and believes that G-d revealed Himself at Mt. Sinai 3899 years ago at an eyewitnessed event before over half a million people who heard the Commandments. He believes that G-d gave the Torah, both the written and oral laws to the Israelites with the command to observe and perform these Commandments or Laws. The religious Jew affiliates with an orthodox synagogue, prays three times a day, and observes as many of the Commandments as he can. He attends synagogue on the Sabbath and holidays. He eats kosher food, and wears the same clothing as non-Jews, since there is no law against doing this.

The ultraorthodox Jew has the same beliefs as the religious or orthodox Jew, but he may observe the 613 Commandments in a stricter manner. He sets himself apart from other Jews and non-Jews by wearing a long black coat, a wide brimmed black hat (even in summer) and a white shirt opened at the collar without a necktie. He may have long ear locks. The black coat costume which he wears does not necessarily mean that he is more learned or more observant than the average religious or orthodox Jew. He forms a very tiny minority in Israel, but his influence is felt because this is the sect that may stone automobiles if they travel on the Sabbath, or they may cast derogatory remarks at Jewish girls who dress immodestly in shorts and bras, and stroll through the geographic areas where these ultras live, such as the Mea Shearim area of Jerusalem.

The secular Jew denies the Revelation at Sinai and does not attend or affiliate with a synagogue. He may or may not believe in G-d, but does not adhere to the 613 commandments, since he believes the Torah was written by various historians through the centuries with no connection to G-d. Since the Jewish religion is of little interest to him, his objective is to uphold the State of Israel as a cultural, non-religious, national, western-type democracy wherein the Jewish religion is anathema with regard to the state. He considers the State of Israel as a national state, like any other state in the world, where the Jews are a cultural entity, and the Jewish religion is a non-essential burden.

The reform and reconstructionist Jew believes in G-d, affiliates with a temple, but like the secular Jew denies the validity of the divine revelation at Sinai. By vote of a committee the reform leadership selects those laws which they think appropriate for the century or age in which they live, and discards those Laws which they feel are inappropriate for the times. Their rationale for doing this is based on the belief that if man, not G-d wrote the Torah or 613 biblical laws, then man, meaning the committee of reform rabbis in each generation, can change them to suit local conditions. As a result of this reasoning they have eliminated the Laws regarding Kosher food, work or riding on the Sabbath, and many other regulations which differentiate the orthodox Jew from the reform and reconstructionist.

The conservative Jew affiliates with a conservative synagogue, believes in G-d and is in a perpetual state of confusion as he vacillates between orthodoxy and reform since his leadership has been unable to define exactly what he is.

Modern or political secular Zionism arose for two reasons: to bring the Jew out of the physical danger of the Exile as a haven of refuge and to create a new and totally different kind of Jew, a Jew who would no longer be tied to the laws and rules and regulations of religion.

For 2,000 years the Jewish people were clearly identified as a religious nation. A gentile who wished to "become Jewish" certainly did not do the same as anyone wishing to become English or French or German. He had to join the Jewish religion by converting. There was no such thing as a secular Jew. If the Jews were a nation, a people, that was only because of the Torah of Judaism.

And all that changed with the rise of modern political Zionism whose aim was to make the Jew like many other peoples of the earth. The father of political Zionism Theodore Herzl had no positive religious Jewish feelings. It was the shock of the Dreyfus trial in Paris in which he saw civilized, liberal France, rage with anti-Jewish passions. The great irony is that the father of modern Zionism was turned into an active Jew not by a Jew, but by the Jew-haters, not through Judaism, but through the gentile. Herzl rejected the Hebrew faith, the Hebrew language, and was prepared to accept Uganda as a Jewish State.

Gershon Shocken, editor of the Israeli paper Haaretz, and himself a secular Zionist delivered a paper in 1984 in which he said: "Zionism in Eastern Europe was, perhaps first and foremost, a rebellion against the Jewish religion. They wanted to uproot it so that there would be no trace of it in the new Jewish society they wished to create."

Chaim Weizman, one of the leaders of modern Zionism, and the first President of Israel warned against any effort to attract religious Jews into the modern Zionist camp: "This will lead straight to catastrophe," he said. If there is anything in Judaism that has become intolerable and incomprehensible to the best of Jewish youth, it is the pressure to equate its essence with the religious formalism of the orthodox. Jewish youth, he added, could be saved through Zionism and a return to Jewish culture, "but Jewish culture should no longer be confused with Jewish religious worship."

Religion, tradition, G-d, were no longer the relevant aspects of the Jewish people. The new Jew, the Hebrew, would be freed of all religious restraints and would be like all the other nations.

The leading American Zionist, Justice Louis Brandeis, a member of the U.S. Supreme Court, was a non-believer who conceived of Zionism as an ideal that would replace the Jewish religion. Jewish nationalism was to Brandeis "an attractive substitute for the Jewish religion."

The early Zionists were non-religious socialists who emigrated from Poland, Russia, Roumania and other countries. Ben Gurion was among those that set up a state that duplicated the impossible bureaucracy which existed in their countries, and this bureaucracy is still in existence today, tying up the free flow of progress, such as exists no where else in the world. That Israel has achieved all that it has in the past 40 years plus winning all the wars is obviously a miracle—a happening outside the natural law.

According to Torah law the stranger who happens to live in the land, like the Arab, must not be ill-treated, or oppressed. He should be treated kindly, his sick should be healed, he is entitled to personal rights, economic, cultural and social rights, but not the right to say anything about the structure or character of the State of Israel. In 1987, the Israel consular representative in Atlanta, Georgia is an Arab. Is this normal or does the Israeli government need a national psychiatrist?

It has been estimated that if unlimited United States visas were available half of all the secular Israelis would emigrate to the U.S. The secular Zionist dream has fallen victim to a bankrupt educational system and the values of a state that is not religiously oriented, but a Hebrew-speaking Portugal seeking to be a caricature of the United States.

Because of the secular nature of those running the Israeli Government the land now wallows in gentile films—the worst of Hollywood and Paris, and televised pornography direct from the depraved Madison Avenue dens of iniquity. The modesty of holiness is contemptuously abandoned and the nation degenerates in the nakedness of the culture of Broadway and 42nd Street in New York and the Pigalle in Paris.

I interviewed secular Israelis, religious Israelis, Christian Arabs and Moslim Arabs and found an interesting cross section of opinion.

The Arabs in Israel are caught between the jaws of a vice. Those who are peaceful, not terrorists, and who prefer to live in Israel rather than the dictatorship which exists across the river in Jordan, resent the terrorists who ultimately make their lives miserable. Each Arab must carry an identify card, actually a small passport-size booklet. These booklets indicate the area in which the Arab lives, such as Jerusalem, Tel Aviv, Hebron, Haifa, etc. An Arab walking the streets of Israel can be stopped four or five times within a two-block area by Israeli soldiers or police, his identity card examined, and his name written down in the policeman's record book. There is an important reason for this. Should a bomb explode in a supermarket or theatre or should an Israeli soldier be stabbed to death every Arab on police record books is rounded up, arrested, and given the third degree as to his guilt or innocence in the bombing or stabbing. Meanwhile all streets and neighborhoods are blocked off by police so that no one can enter or leave and this blockade may go on for days.

Not every Arab is a terrorist, yet the innocent ones suffer the public embarrassment and intimidation incurred by the few terrorists.

Israeli plain clothes security men as well as uniformed soldiers and police can sniff out an Arab youth who may dress and look exactly like an Israeli, and they seldomly mistake the identification.

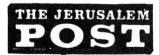

Friday, July 24, 1987   The Jerusalem Post

Moslem Arabs living in Israel are no friend of the state. In a crisis they would be an overwhelming fifth column who would join ranks with their Moslem brethern since a war against Israel is considered a Jihad or holy war as willed by Allah.

The Kach party, represented in the Knesset by Rabbi Meir Kahane, advocates that Arabs can remain in Israel so long as they agree not to demand national rights, meaning they accept their status as non-voting citizens who have no say in the government, and cannot serve in the I.D.F. or Israel Defense Forces. This reasoning by Kach will certainly not remove the resentment which the Arabs harbor against the Israeli Government, nor will it remove the threat of a fifth column in the event of war by the 400 million Arabs which surround Israel from Egypt to Syria.

Secular Jews, those who may believe in G-d, but scoff at the concept that the Torah was given by G-d in an eye-witnessed event at Mt. Sinai, have two different problems on their hands. They do not observe the Sabbath. They do not attend the synagogue, and they may intermarry with an Arab girl if they leave Israel and get married in Cyprus. Yet they may have deep feelings for the land of Israel since they were born here; this is their land, and they resent the Arab presence because the Arab is a constant threat to their lives.

The other problem is his religious Jewish brother, especially the "black coats," the ones whose ear locks dangle down to the chin, who wear long black coats and wide-brimmed, black hats and white shirts open at the neck without ties even on the sweltering days of midsummer.

The majority of religious Jews in Israel are not of the "black coat" variety. The "black coats" are comparatively few and are conspicuous only because of their contrast with western style clothing, but they are a distinct minority. Most of the religious Jews do not wear "black coats" nor do they have dangling ear locks. On the Sabbath they go to the synagogues dressed no differently from American religious Jews attending synagogues in Baltimore, New York or Los Angeles.

The secular Jew must serve in the Army and perform a month of national guard service each year until the age of 55. The religious Jew who has been studying in a Yeshiva is exempted from this. The secular Jew resents this.

The secular Jew does not resent the Arab as much as he resents his brother, the religious Jew. The religious Jew through his power in the government, has stopped all buses from operating on the Sabbath in Jerusalem. However, buses still run in Haifa on the Sabbath. The religious Jew publicly criticizes his secular brother because of the immorality and pornography in films, magazines, and television. The secular Jew tells the religious Jew to mind his own business, that Israel is a western-type democracy and a citizen can do whatever he wishes within the law. The religious Jew says Israel is a Jewish state and only Jews should vote and only Jews should serve in the Knesset. The religious Jew says since Israel is a Jewish state it cannot be a democracy. It is a state to be run only by

Jews. The secular Jew is more on the side of the Arabs than his nemesis, the religious Jew. And the religious Jew in the Knesset works hard to institute laws that uphold the Torah which the secular Jew does not observe.

The infighting between the two Jewish factions has repercussions within families. An example: A secular, successful Jewish businessman has a son who came under the influence of a "black coat" religious Jew. The son permitted his hair to grow into long ear locks, he purchased a black coat and a wide brimmed hat, entered a Yeshiva or religious school and married a religious girl. He then refused to eat in his father's secular Jewish house. The father disowned him, and refuses to see his five grandchildren because the son became too Jewish for the secular Jewish father and mother. The father and mother were embarrassed, for what would their secular circle of friends think of them harboring a son with earlocks and a black coat? This is a true story that I personally witnessed.

One can deduce from this the resentment that secular Jews harbor for their religious brothers. This resentment among secular Jews for their more orthodox children has created such tensions that an organization has arisen in Israel of secular parents against what they see as brainwashing and seducing their children into cults.

The secular Jews who run the Israeli Government are worried and quite concerned about a problem which seems almost unbelievable. Secular Israelis are leaving Israel in droves for the United States and other Western countries. Secular Israeli women are having abortions. The only influx of Jews from the West is of religious Jews, and the religious Jews are producing the babies in Israel. The problem: if this keeps up the majority of the Jews in Israel will be orthodox and this would be calamitous to the government. Instead of being afraid of the Arab population explosion, their main fear is the orthodox Jewish population explosion.

The Arabs, on the other hand, hate the Jews with a passion. Every Arab I interviewed is riddled with hate, and believes what he reads in his pro-PLO, Arabic newspapers. He reads that the Jews, by force of arms, stole Palestine which they renamed Israel, from the poor Arabs. The historic truth of how the United Nations voted to establish a Jewish state where both Arabs and Jews could live in peace is ignored. The Arabs were given the entire West Bank and Gaza, and the Jews through the Jewish National Fund, bought and paid for every inch of ground they occupied in Israel. The Arabs opposed the vote of the United Nations and went to war against Israel in 1948, killed over 6,000 Jews and lost the war.

And today in Israel, Arab after Arab told me Israel stole the country from them, and that eventually they will kill every Jew and get their country back.

The big lie that Hitler used so effectively in Germany is being used here in Israel by the Arabs. And the Israeli Government does nothing about this. It permits the Arabs to read this inciting propaganda in the Arabic newspaper, while Israeli soldiers are knifed or shot in ambush. A typical event occurred in Gaza on Monday, August 8, 1987 while I was there. An Israeli soldier on duty in Gaza was shot in the head in broad daylight as a terrorist act. The Arabic newspapers reported that the Israeli soldier who was shot had forced a coke bottle up the rectum of an Arab child and that the soldier was being paid back. The truth was, the soldier who was shot happened to be in his Jeep, caught in a traffic jam and was the random target for terrorists looking for a victim. The dead soldier, age 22, was in charge of the police detachment in Gaza. The coke bottle story was a falsehood, and this is what Israeli authorities permit the Arabs to read in the name of "democracy".

The Israeli government is obviously in dire need of a psychiatric couch. It seems to enjoy doing itself in. Every Moslem Arab quoted the Koran "that there is no place in this world for the Jews, and that ultimately the Jews will all be killed." As one East Jerusalem Arab shopkeeper put it, "The Koran says that even the stones shall cry out against the Jews," and that not one Jew will be left alive in Palestine.

After a thorough investigation of the political situation, and innumerable interviews with both Israeli Jews, secular and religious, and with Christian and Moslem Arabs, I am still confused about this remarkable little country which made the word miracle a veritable reality.

CHAPTER VI

THE BEDOUIN TRIBES OF ISRAEL

The Bedouins are tribes of people who live in the deserts of southern Israel. How they survive in a waterless, hot desert was so intriguing to me that I investigated some aspects of their life style.

They live in large, sprawling tents, the cloth of which they weave themselves, from black goat hair, since the hair swells in the rain which keeps the inside of the tent dry. Their clothes are almost identical to those worn by our Biblical forefathers. Their daily bread is unleavened matzo. Their tent is called a Soukka, which Jews dwell in one week each autumn to commemorate dwelling in Soukkas during the 40 years of wandering in the wilderness after receiving the Torah.

The Bedouins trace their origins to the nomads of the Arabian peninsula from about the 14th century. They came in small groups, some fleeing drought and others from enemies.

The Bedouins have divided up the Sinai desert into tribal areas which are unmarked by any visible boundaries. The limited water sources, the pasture for their goats and sheep, and the right to cultivate the land belong exclusive to the tribe possessing it. The area around Beersheba, for example, is staked off by the Azazma tribe. Their tents can be seen from all the highways leading to Beersheba. The tribes near Jerusalem are known as the Tiyaha tribe and their tents are visible on the road to the Dead Sea from Jerusalem.

The affairs of a tribe are managed by a chief known as a Shaykh. He is usually a charismatic individual and is elected by the adult males. The chief exercises his authority only by persuasion, since the Bedouins are characteristically quite independent. If the tribe grows too large they may split up into new groups with new chiefs. The Tiyaha tribe now has seventeen chiefs.

The pursuit of the Bedouins is raising livestock, especially the black goat, sheep and camels. The camel provides hair for the tent, milk for the family and for the campfire. Camels were created for the desert. They can graze on thorns, and dried-out bushes. Their bodies conserve water and their blood preserves its consistency even when they are dehydrated. The camel can fluctuate his body temperature by 46 degrees Fahrenheit each day in order to withstand the hot desert sun and the cold nights. Throughout the year the Bedouin migrates according to a pattern based on seasonal needs such as water wells and springs. After the autumn rains he leaves his water sources to let new grasses grow there, for his flocks and herds will need them the next summer. Every year Bedouins plough a patch of land with camels hitched to an ancient style plough. They get a crop every four or five years which is usually too thin to harvest with a sickle. Each stalk is usually plucked separately by hand. Those Bedouins who live along sea coasts often take to fishing.

Family life among the Bedouins will usually find the men sitting around talking and drinking coffee while the women are away tending the flocks, gathering firewood, tending his children or mending the tent. But the Bedouin family is in the business of raising livestock. The man of the family is the manager, he buys and sells animals, finds new pastures, decides when the family should migrate, and does all the marketing. He is also prepared to fight in order to protect his flocks and the honor of his family.

If a Bedouin wants a wife, he has to buy her, as no bride is obtained free. The price of the bride is calculated in camels. Five to seven camels is considered a fair price for a good woman. Marital links are decided upon by families, family interests taking priority over romantic inclinations. Divorce is quite easy. A displeased husband simple sends his wife back to her family, but he pays for child support. There is no alimony. The Muslim religion allows a Bedouin to have four wives simultaneously. The usual practice is two wives: an older one and a younger one to help with the chores.

The clothing of a Bedouin woman consists of a long dress, veil, a belt and a black shawl to cover her head. Girls start to wear these items at puberty, and any woman wearing less is considered "naked". The man wears a head-kerchief known as a Kufiyya which is held down by a rope known as the Agahl. He also wears a wide-hemmed gown which Bedouins feel is more comfortable than pants.

Bedouins exist on a simple diet that consists of dry bread or pita for breakfast, and fresh bread for lunch. Their supper consists of bread soaked in butter or in a soup made of desert herbs. They bake their own bread on a metal disc called a Saj. The diet may vary with partridge eggs, sour milk, and cheese made from goat's milk. Despite the meager diet they can walk for miles, barefoot over stones, and climb high hills with

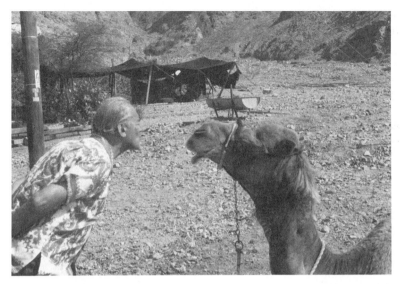

I talk to a friendly camel belonging to the Beduin family who reside in the black goat hair tent in the background.

agility. The lack of Vitamin A in the diet accounts for much night blindness.

To immunize her children against scorpion bites, the mother catches scorpions, burns them, and lets the infant imbibe the ash while nursing. The Bedouins are also fond of burning their aches and pains by a system of cauterization called Kavy, which is a form of desert acupuncture or moxibustion.

Religious belief centers on the one god Allah and his prophet Mohammed. Their practice of the Muslim religion is very unorthodox. One of their main practices is to make visits to the tombs of holy persons and ancestors. There they slaughter a goat as an offering to the Wili, or holy man and ask him to intervene with Allah on behalf of themselves, their children or their livestock. They seek the protection of Allah against drought, floods, wolves, and snakes. They believe that envious people can harm the objects they envy by looking at them. This is called "the evil eye". Bedouins are particularly careful to shield their children and flocks from the glances of unknown persons, and especially cameras.

Dogs are considered impure and should not be petted. Certain bushes or trees in the desert are believed to contain a human spirit and must not be cut or even trimmed. To violate a taboo is to endanger one's health or very life.

The twentieth century is marking the end of Bedouin culture. Modern schools are being set up near the campsites of tribal chiefs, and children are learning to read and write instead of tending their father's goats and sheep. Pick-up trucks are replacing the camel for transportation, and the permanent house is replacing the tent. So much of what I saw among the Bedouins reminded me of the American Indians who are discarding the tepee for houses on the reservations.

CHAPTER VII

DOCTORS MAKE
THE WORST PATIENTS

Retirement is also that time of life when we propose to do all the things we dreamed about doing during the long period of working years. My retirement dream was interrupted while on a trip to California by an ailment which I refused to acknowledge.

It all started on a weekend in California. I was awakened by a painful desire to urinate at about 2 A.M. in a Los Angeles hotel. I tried and tried, leaned against the wall, bore down as much as I was able, but to no avail—the urine would not come forth. I thought my abdomen would burst. I calmed myself. I would just stand there and wait it out. Soon a few drops appeared. Then a thin, weak sporadic stream appeared and the burning and pain which accompanied this painful effort was unbearable. Finally I squeezed out half a glass of urine which was cloudy and streaked with foreign matter and of a foul odor. I collapsed into my bed in a sweat, totally exhausted.

What happened to me? I would call a urologist first thing in the morning.

At 4 A.M. a similar episode occurred. This time I feared standing because of the possibility of fainting, so I knelt on the floor holding a glass to collect the urine which was pressing to be extruded. But something was obstructing its passage. The pain was excruciating. Would I be able to crawl to the telephone to call an ambulance? Soon another two ounces escaped. I could not lift myself into the bed. I lay on the carpeted floor, totally exhausted, and fell asleep for an hour. Again I was awakened with the same intractable pain. I swallowed three Empirin tablets and managed to squeeze out another two ounces.

At 8:30 I phoned a urologist. The pain was somewhat assuaged by the Empirin. I told him I could not see him since I was on my way back to Baltimore, but he did prescribe a urinary analgesic, Azo Gantricin and penicillin. I spent the remainder of the day in bed and the next day flew back to Baltimore.

I made an immediate appointment with Dr. Martin Robbins, Chief of Urology at Baltimore's Sinai Hospital who took my history which I related as follows:

For several years my urinary stream had been decreasing in strength, output, width and length. I attributed this to a natural aging process consistent with a natural enlarging of the prostate gland which most men at age 60 experience. Yearly rectal examinations of my prostate did not reveal any unusual enlargement, some to be sure, but not sufficient to cause any alarming remarks from the lubricated, gloved finger of the examining physician.

During the past six months I began to notice an urgency to urinate when I stepped out of a warm automobile into the cold outside. There was also an urgency to urinate upon standing upright after sitting for a prolonged period. The process of urination to assuage the urgency did not produce a sufficient quantity of urine to justify the intense degree of urgency. And there were many occasions when I had to wait from two to three minutes before the urine began to flow, in non-steady, start and stop spurts. I found myself leaning against the wall for support and many times found it more convenient to sit on the toilet to wait out the urinary flow rather than stand and strain.

My sleep became increasingly interrupted. Sometimes I was awakened two or three times during the night by an urgent, pressing desire to urinate, only to discover that once in the bathroom poised to produce, the urine hesitated to flow and only by patient straining could I relieve myself of this unbearable pressure within my bladder. Each night this occurred I vowed that I would call a urologist in the morning, but the thought of having a cystoscope inserted into me, which I knew he would have to do, deterred me from calling. I had put hundreds of patients to sleep for cystoscopy examinations, and I had seen so many torn prostatic misadventures, prolonged bleeding for days following simple cystoscopic examinations, that the visions of these mishaps happening to me cancelled my nocturnal vows.

I read a book on the prostate by Gilbert Cant. I went to the library and read everything on urinary retention and benign prostatic hypertrophy. I spoke to health fadists who prescribed zinc tablets. I was on mega zinc for six months hoping this would overcome my problem. I stopped drinking coffee, tea, and chocolate beverages, and also alcoholic drinks, all of which were supposed to be guilty of irritating the prostate gland. The visions of the cystoscope entering my body was more unbearable than the discomfort I was forcing myself to endure. I diagnosed my condition as prostatitis and prescribed for myself the same drugs that the California urologist suggested, antibiotics and Azo Gantricin. The acuteness of my discomfort was assuaged for temporary periods by the drugs which fostered false hopes. I began to carry an empty Planters Peanut jar in my car to relieve myself when urgency overcame me in my automobile. I became expert at urinating while driving my car. The peanut jar was always of adequate capacity since the amount of urine expelled was always of such a small volume. Some mornings I awakened to find that I had leaked urine into my pajamas. Yet when I arose to urinate the quantity was of such a small volume that I became puzzled as to the cause of the leakage.

The acute pain finally drove me to phone Dr. Robbins but I did so with great reluctance. I was certain that the prostate had suddenly swollen in the area of my urethra and that the ingestion of some magical drugs that Dr. Robbins might be familiar with would alleviate my condition. I presented all these facts in typewritten form to Dr. Robbins.

His first remark after reading this history was "Sylvan, take this bottle into the next room and pee in it, then bring it right back into my office." With much effort, accompanied with severe pain I oozed out about an ounce of cloudy urine. I handed the bottle to Dr. Robbins. He looked at it and said: "Sylvan, your urine is grossly infected. Remove your pants and shorts and lie on this table. I did so. He placed his hand on my pubic bone and gently palpated my abdomen, going up slowly toward my umbilicus. He said with great alarm: "Sylvan, you have exactly one hour to go home, get your things together, and report to the admitting office of Sinai Hospital. I'm admitting you as an emergency patient in acute urinary retention. As soon as you are in your room I'll arrive and catheterize you since your bladder is bulging with over a quart of urine that can't get out. The catheter will remain in your bladder for about five days, you'll be on antibiotics, when your urine cultures are negative I'll cystoscope you and then I'll decide what is to be done thereafter."

I could not believe my own ears. I protested: "Can't you treat me medically? Why must I enter the hospital?" Dr. Robbins became impatient with me and said: "This is a life-threatening situation. If that infected urine backs up into your kidneys you can die." That's all I had to hear, but I only half believed that I could be retaining a quart of urine, since at the moment I had no desire to urinate.

I dashed home and packed an overnight bag. I arrived at the hospital and was admitted with the usual question: "Who is your nearest of kin that we can call in an emergency?" I was taken to my room. I undressed, got into my robe and awaited the arrival of Dr. Robbins. While waiting I thought that I would fool him. I went into the bathroom and urinated all I could squeeze out of my bladder, which was about two ounces. I'd prove to him that there was no urine in my bladder and that hospitalizing me was unnecessary, and that he simply missed the diagnosis. I just could not visualize 32 ounces of urine in my bladder.

Soon Dr. Robbins came hurrying down the corridor and entered my room with a sterile catheter tray. I did not inform him that I had "emptied" my bladder just minutes ago.

He directed me to lie on my back. He placed a large square basin between my legs, he cleansed my genitals, lubricated the tip of a rubber, foley catheter, and inserted it into my bladder. As it passed through the swollen prostate and past my internal sphincter it felt like a searing, white flame within my pelvis. This lasted only a moment. What happened after that I could not believe even though I was seeing the dramatic deluge with my own eyes.

Urine was pouring out of that catheter in such a rush that it overshot the basin. Not only did it fill the basin which held a quart, but it partially filled a second basin with cloudy, infected urine. In all, over a quart of urine poured out of me and the bulging tummy that I had been wanting to reduce by sit-ups and other exercises disappeared as suddenly as a pregnant abdomen flattens when the baby is delivered.

I was speechless, flabergasted, and I felt so stupid at my abysmal ignorance since I should have known better, having been administering anesthesia for many urologists for so many years. But I suppose that on a subconscious level I just did not want to face the truth which necessitated any instrumentation on this part of my anatomy.

Dr. Robbins informed me that I might be in the hospital for at least two weeks. That the foley catheter would remain in my bladder in order to drain it until the urine cultures were negative and at that time he would do the thing I dreaded most—the cystoscopy in order to make a proper diagnosis as to how to prevent this acute condition from reoccurring.

I was so embarrassed by my massive denial that I answered: "Yes sir, anything you say." He instructed me to drink oceans of water and that I would be on Ampicillin every six hours around the clock till further notice. My foley catheter was connected to a plastic reservoir bag which was attached to the side of my bed. He left the room and said he would see me in the morning. It was 3 P.M. on Friday, January 11, 1980. My room was a marvel of electrical gagetry. I could open and close the drapes by electricity. Suspended over my bed was a spring loaded electric arm with a battery of switches that operated not only the curtains, but the electric lights in the room, as well as the TV set, plus an electric all button for the nurse. Other switches operated the all-electric bed.

After investigating my surroundings I was relieved that I was at last having this long neglected condition treated. I was irritated at the sudden interruption of my multitude of activities. I reached for the phone, informed my family and friends as to my whereabouts, and so began my hospital sojourn for intensive treatment of a condition known as acute urinary retention caused by BPH, or benign prostatic hypertrophy.

I glanced at the plastic bag attached to the bedside. It was filling up with cloudy urine. I watched afternoon television for awhile. If retirement was ever implied being condemned to viewing daytime TV then I was certain that retirement could become worse punishment than being imprisoned by this indwelling catheter and plastic bag. Daytime television with its soap operas, give away games, and incessant boring commercials could be worse than a jail term. I tried to read. The catheter was not comfortable. I could not concentrate.

After lying on my back for what seemed to be a prolonged period, I attempted to turn to change my position and then the spasm occurred. No one had warned me about the insufferable pain caused by a bladder spasm which is initiated by the bladder clamping down on the inflated foley balloon inside the bladder. The bladder interprets the balloon as a bolus of urine and constricts against it in an attempt to expel it. The pain is absolutely excruciating. Fortunately it lasts only two or three minutes and then evaporates much like a labor pain. In order to avoid triggering the spasm the tendency is to lie unmoving in bed. This is also self defeating since buttocks, legs and back begin to numb from the pressure of lying still. But move I must. Then a bright thought entered my mind. I'd ask the nurse for some pain pills, wait till they became effective, then I could move and the pain of bladder spasms would probably not be so severe.

I pushed the red, nurse-call button.

Over a hidden loudspeaker in my room a kind voice answered: "May I help you?" What efficiency, I thought. I couldn't get over how swiftly the response was to my electrified call button. "I'm having considerable pain from bladder spasms. May I have pain pills immediately, please?" "Right away" came the reply.

But the reply was far swifter than the service. Twenty minutes later I pushed the button and repeated my request. "Right away" again came the reply. But no nurse, no pain pills, and I was now in my third spasm and this last spasm came spontaneously without being initiated by body movement. Again I pushed the red button. The answer was immediate, "May I

help you?" "Yes, damn it", I answered, "but if you do not bring me some
pain pills immediately I'm going to phone Dr. Robbins directly, then I'll
call President Carter, and also the S.P.C.M.—the society for the preven-
tion of cruelty to man!"

Thirty minutes after that last call, and about an hour after the initial
call I received two tablets of Tylenol #3. This combination of Tylenol and
codeine had a remarkable effect and it lasted about three hours. I could
now turn and twist, I could feel the spasms occurring, but the painful
aspect had been attenuated. I was not about to depend upon the whims of a
busy nursing staff to bring me future doses of Tylenol two hours after I
demanded it, so I phoned my office, had my associate write a prescription
for the drug, had my secretary bring it to the hospital, and I hid it safely,
but conveniently in my night table. I was now free to take pain relievers at
will, and free of bladder spasms.

I was drinking copious quantities of water and my urine bag bulged
accordingly. The food served to me in bed wasn't too bad and a five mg.
tablet of Valium at bedtime permitted easy sleep in an otherwise noisy
environment.

Five days later my urine had cleared, my bladder was shrinking back to
normal size, I had undergone chest x-rays, a battery of blood tests, and an
intravenous pyelogram. Dr. Robbins announced that tomorrow he would
inspect the inside of my bladder with a cystoscope—the instrument I
dreaded most. After the cystoscopy Dr. Robbins would decide what was to
be done to prevent a recurrence of my problem. I pointed out to Dr.
Robbins that since I was an anesthesiologist and knew the inherent dangers
of total general anesthesia, especially for minor procedures such as cystoscopy, that I did not want to go to sleep, neither did I want to receive a
spinal anesthetic. He assured me that I would feel no pain. He would
install Xylocaine first, then wait five minutes before inserting the cystoscope, and, in addition, he would inject 10 mg. of Valium intravenously.
He assured me that I would feel no pain.

The dreaded morning for cystoscopy arrived. An orderly placed his
litter next to my bed and had me slide on to it. My private nurse helped
me change into an open back operating room gown. A pillow was placed
under my head, the side guards of the litter were raised and the long ride
down twisting corridors and elevators began.

I noticed the recessed fluorescent lights in the ceilings of the hospital
corridors as well as the safety fire sprinkling systems and other items that
individuals not on their backs seldom notice. The cystoscopy section of
Sinai Hospital appeared to be half a block long. I was parked against a

wall, lined up with many other patients awaiting their turn in what I thought was this chamber of silent misery, the chamber of searing, white hot flaming torture that I experienced when the foley catheter first entered my bladder. Dr. Robbins appeared in his green surgical scrub suit, several sizes too large, from one of the many doorways opening into this long hallway of unhappiness. He leaned on my litter guard rails and said: "Sylvan, I think you're going to be all right. Just relax. You'll have no discomfort and I'll take good care of you and the entire examination won't take over about five minutes." He squeezed my arm for reassurance. Dr. Robbins did not realize, I'm certain, how much I needed those kind words and the friendly squeeze of my arm to reassure me. It had a greater effect upon me than a shot of morphine.

Soon my time came.

I was wheeled into one of the many mysterious doorways leading off the hallway into a cystoscopy room. There was the familiar, hard cystoscopy table with knee supports, an X-ray tube overhead with thick high tension wires extruding from it. My legs were suspended in the knee supports and a friendly nurse cleansed my genital area with a warm antiseptic solution which was very considerate since I had seen so many patients flinch and draw back when cold solutions were poured over this area of the body.

Dr. Robbins strapped my right arm to an extended arm board, inserted a 21-gauge needle into my vein, and quickly injected 5 mg. of Valium. My private nurse held my hand. The Valium did very little for me. After several minutes the remaining 5 mg. of Valium was injected through the indwelling needle. I now had received a total of 10 mg. of Valium. I saw the ceiling tiles and studied their design. One of the fluorescent tubes was dimmer than the other. How many other unfortunate patients had stared up at this ceiling? I suddenly realized that my anxiety and apprehension had vanished and somehow I was simply focused on the square acoustical blocks of the ceiling design. I studied the ceiling with a peculiar compulsion and felt as if all other thoughts, fears and anxieties had vanished and the only important object in the world was the design of the ceiling and the dim fluorescent light bulb.

Suddenly Dr. Robbins said to me: "Sylvan, we're all finished. The cystoscope is out and your fresh foley catheter is in and the operation is over."

"But I did not feel you start," I protested. "I was staring at the ceiling. It's impossible. What time is it? I felt absolutely nothing. You're joking with me. How did you insert that cystoscope without my knowing it?"

And then I realized for the first time that I was asking the same unbelieving questions patients ask me after giving them Valium for the filling and extraction of teeth. They insist, as I insisted, that I was awake and aware of every second of elapsed time and that never for a moment was I unaware of my surroundings. But what happened to me was what I had imposed on about 20,000 patients over a period of 20 years. But I had never achieved this state of complete amnesia with Valium alone since my dosage range of the drug was always less than 10 mg. I supplemented Valium with a micro-dose of Brevital or Pentothal which assured amnesia. In my case the 10 mg. of Valium was apparently sufficient not only to block my memory of the entire event, but it had effectively and efficiently stopped my internal physiological clock so that I had no concept of the passage of the previous 20 minutes. That was the time it took to instill Xylocaine in my bladder, insert the cystoscope, distend my bladder with saline and inspect all aspects of the cavernous, mysterious wonderland which, when in health, operates automatically without a conscious thought from the brain-control centers.

My nurse informed me that when the Xylocaine was instilled into my bladder to numb the passageway prior to inserting the cystoscope, I grimmaced and squeezed her hand. She asked me how I felt and I answered that it burned. When the cystoscope was inserted I grimaced again in pain and kept looking at the ceiling. She further informed me that Dr. Robbins leisurely explored the mountains and valleys of my bladder's interior, and even stopped for awhile to take an emergency phone call. All the while I answered questions when presented to me, and my nurse herself was not aware of the depth of the stage of amnesia, of forgetfulness, of the fact that my internal clock mechanism had ceased functioning which effectively obliterated my conscious concept of the passage of time. As far as I was concerned I was still studying the ceiling tiles, the rectangular X-ray tube and the one, dim, fluorescent light bulb.

The conversations, questions and my answers, and Dr. Robbins' phone call, the several jokes told which are popular in most operating rooms were impinging on my ear drums, causing a reaction in my speech center so that I laughed, spoke, and even joked along with the assistants. but the memory bank in my brain was severed as surely as were the painful impulses coursing up my spinal cord from the stretch and water distension of my bladder during the cystoscopic instrumentation. Nothing of this 20-minute episode was recorded in my memory. And so thorough and complete was the chemical severence of my memory from the effects of the Valium that it was as if nothing had happened. Yet it all happened since I have observed this phenomenon in thousands of my own patients. After all these years of imposing this aura of amnesia without the dangers of unconsciousness in the form of general anesthesia in my own patients, it was the first time I had ever experienced it myself under conditions of real fear, deep anxiety, and intense apprehension. The totality of the obliteration of these miserable pitch-forked demons aroused in me a greater appreciation of what patients undergo, and more important, of the role of mercy I have played during the past two decades.

Dr. Robbins informed me that two days hence he would have to perform a transurethral resection or a T.U.R. of a portion of my hypertrophic prostate gland in order to carve out a wider, more normal passage for my urine. He assured me that after the T.U.R., instead of urinating a thin, sickly stream requiring minutes to empty my bladder, I would be able to urinate like a cow urinating on a flat rock with all the rush, ease, force and gusto of a fire hose.

Back to my room again for two days. My bladder was still draining through the foley catheter, but the spasms had all disappeared. There was no pain or bleeding after the cystoscopy and my urine took on the appearance of fine vintage *vin blanc.*

My hospital room was meanwhile filling up with a multitude of floral decorations, baskets of fruit, balloons for the sick, and a myriad of get-well cards, many with bizarre instructions on how to keep the nurses happy, and some of them threatening to surreptitiously tug at my catheter while I was asleep.

The day of my T.U.R. operation arrived.

The anesthesiologist had visited me the night before and very modestly asked me to write my own prescription for the spinal anesthetic since we, as well as the surgeon, agreed that spinal was best for this particular operation. I did insist, however, that he inject some ephedrine intramuscularly about five minutes prior to injecting the spinal Pontocaine in order to stabilize my blood pressure.

The next day I was wheeled down the long, long corridors to the same cystoscopy area where the T.U.R. was to be performed. Having had the experience of severe bladder spasms for several days from a small, rubber foley catheter, I imagine that the deep pelvic pain from an electrical dissection of my prostate, plus an even larger post operative foley catheter with a balloon twice the size would involve pain of an unbearable nature once the spinal wore off.

I wrote a note to the surgeon which I handed to him in the operating room requesting that I be given the right to choose my own post-operative, pain-relief medication depending upon how I felt. The note read as follows:

"POST OP ORDERS FOR SYLVAN SHANE

Patient to have the choice of the following drugs to be administered at *HIS* discretion:

DILAUDID 1 or 2 mg P.O.
q 3 to 4 h PRN for pain

OR

TYLENOL #3 P.O. q 3 to 4 h
PRN for pain"

Dr. Robbins handed the note back to me with the following notation:

"You cook in your kitchen and I'll
cook in mine."
(Signed) THE CHEF

Dr. Robbins assured me that the post-operative orders as as I had written them were satisfactory with him, and with that the anesthesiologist proceeded with the spinal.

Although I have administered several thousand spinal anesthetics during my 18 years as an anesthesiologist, I have personally never been on the receiving end of a spinal needle. It was quite an experience.

During his pre-operative visit the night before surgery, the anesthesiologist described what he thought was the proper management of the spinal. He would first give me 500 cc. of lactated Ringers solution, very rapidly, prior to injecting the spinal anesthetic solution, Pontocaine, in order to avert any fall in blood pressure which normally occurs after the spinal anesthetic is injected.

I objected to this. I suggested that in my experience intramuscular ephedrine, 25 mg., would be a more certain guarantee against a fall in blood pressure. The anesthesiologist persisted in his belief based on his experience and I reluctantly agreed. I also suggested that he administer no more than 6 mg. of Pontocaine. He insisted on 8 mg. Again I reluctantly agreed, even though I felt that the dose was excessive for a pelvic operation in a sixty-year-old man.

I emphasized the fact that under no circumstances did I want to be rendered unconscious, and that I had selected spinal anesthesia in order to avoid general-sleep anesthesia with its far greater risks. It has been estimated that one person in approximately 10,000 rendered unconscious from general anesthesia will never wake up. The cause of this is unknown. The study was conducted under auspices of the Massachusetts General Hospital after surveying all anesthetics administered in about 50 university hospitals in the United States. Eliminated from the study were patients who died of severe blood loss, misdiagnosis, surgical error, and cardiovascular pathology. The deaths occurred in otherwise health patients.

My emphasis on no sleep I felt was adequately understood by the anesthesiologist.

An intravenous line was established in my right arm and 500 cc. of lactated Ringer's solution began to infuse. I was instructed to sit upright on the operating table. My back was asepticized with Betadene solution. The spinal tap was made and I was surprised to discover how painless it was. As the needle punctured my dura I felt a slight dull ache which was momentary. The anesthesiologist supported me in this upright position for a minute and then had me lie flat on my back with a pillow under my head.

At first a warm sensation crept over my lower extremities. It began to creep upwards. Soon I was unable to move my legs. I mentally gave the command to my legs to move, but my legs refused to obey. The numb feeling continued to creep higher and higher. With my left hand I began pinching my thigh. The skin felt as foreign as if I were pinching the nurse.

I became somewhat agitated when the level of the spinal crept above my umbilicus. Soon it was at my mid-chest then my nipple line. I called this high level to the anesthesiologist's attention, but he kept writing in his little black book and paid no attention to this unnecessary high level. The higher the level of spinal paralysis the more severe is the possible fall in blood pressure since ascending segments of the autonomic nervous system, which are instrumental in maintaining blood pressure, are, one after another rendered inoperative. In addition, as the spinal level ascends, segments of the intercostal muscles which are involved in respiration become paralyzed making it increasingly more difficult to breathe.

When paralysis reached my nipple line, which was at least nine inches above where the spinal should have stopped, I became quite agitated since I knew it should not have progressed above my umbilicus. I could easily detect the creeping by pinching my left side. Soon I felt as if there was a 50-pound weight on my chest and I found it difficult to breathe.

The anesthesiologist could have averted this entire upward creeping episode by simply tilting the operating table in a foot-down position known technically as the reverse Trendelenberg position which would cause the heavier than spinal fluid Pontocaine anesthetic to flow down my spine rather than upwards towards my head. But he was too occupied with his little black book to heed my warnings. When he finished writing in his black book he bestirred himself to rise up out of his chair and place an oxygen mask on my face to facilitate breathing, since at this time both my finger nails and lips had a bluish, cyanotic hue, and the operation had not even begun.

The orderly meanwhile had placed my legs up in stirrups and commenced to asepticize the operative area.

The anesthesiologist, a very friendly colleague of mine for many years, being aware of my agitation because of the unnecessary high level of the spinal and my difficulty in breathing, asked me if I would like a drug to help alleviate my apprehension. My confidence in this man, waning by the moment, I decided to leave nothing to his judgment, and inquired as to what drug he had in mind. He said: "Tell you what. I'll inject the drug and see if you can tell me what it is."

Remembering my emphasis and his promise during his pre-operative visit the evening before concerning my absolute insistence on not being rendered unconscious, I said with some hesitation, "Go ahead, I'll see if I can identify it."

With that he injected a drug into the intravenous tubing which I failed to identify, but it did abolish all my apprehension and I felt quite relieved and delightfully spaced out. My private nurse who stood beside me on the left side of the operating table held the oxygen mask on my face.

For no reason at all, since I was now quite calm, the anesthesiologist said to me: "Now I'm going to inject another drug. See if you can tell what it is." Before I could object (and I felt so good from the previous drug that it made no difference one way or another) he injected it. Soon I was much farther out into outer space.

Again he said to me: "Now see if you can identify this drug." He injected another drug, and I cannot remember what this drug did.

My nurse informed me that he repeated this questioning a fourth time, and injected still another drug, and this time I was rendered unconscious! The drug he injected this time was Sodium Pentothal. I was now under total general anesthesia, a state that I neither gave permission to impose, and a state against which the anesthesiologist promised he would refrain from inducing.

My blood pressure began to fall. His theory of a rapid infusion of intravenous Ringer's solution did not prove sound, and he was forced to inject ephedrine to raise my pressure up to normal as I had suggested the night before.

The next day I obtained a copy of the anesthesia record and was appalled at the utter lack of judgment displayed by this man whom I thought would care for me as a friend. The following are the drugs and the dosages he injected into my veins:

The first drug which spaced me out was Nembutal. He injected twice the dose necessary for a 60-year-old. He injected 50 mg. Upon this overdose he injected the following drugs which were absolutely unnecessary and proved harmful since these drugs are known to augment a falling blood pressure:

> Nisentil (a powerful narcotic) 7 mg.
> Valium (a tranquilizer) 5 mg.
> Pentothal (an anesthetic) 50 mg.

There was no reason on earth for the injection of all these potent drugs, and especially the Pentothal which rendered me unconscious. My body was so numb from the spinal that the surgeon could have cut me in half and I would not have felt it.

The *coup de grace* was, of course, the Pentothal, which rendered me unconscious for the duration of the operation. This was a breach of professional ethics, and an example of the poorest judgement I have ever experienced in 20 years of working in the field of medical anesthesia.

When I inspected my anesthesia chart the next day I also discovered a neat cover up. My blood pressure which fell to 80 systolic (as observed by my nurse in attendance) was not recorded on the anesthesia record. A clear indication of the guilt of this man whom I thought was my friend. I also discovered that he had given me 10 mg. of Pontocaine instead of the 8 mg. we argued about.

I began to awaken in the recovery room where I could feel my feet beginning to move. After a short sojourn in recovery I was taken back to my room where I remained flat for eight hours to prevent post-spinal headache. I kept feeling my thighs which felt like that of a stranger and not my own. Three hours later the spinal wore off but the rectal area was the last to release the spinal's numbing grip. This area was numb for five hours.

In my bladder was a firm, foley catheter attached again to a urine drainage bag, but this foley was less flexible and much larger in size. It appeared as if it was the diameter of a dime and I wondered how I could have been stretched to that severe extent to get such a gigantic tube within me. I felt as the newly-delivered mother must feel when her new-born is presented to her and she contemplates the size of the infant's head and wonders how that gigantic head ever exited from her body.

There seemed to be no pain from the operative site once the spinal wore off, but the foley catheter became my nemesis. I was surprised at the total lack of post-operative pain and also the lack of bladder spasms. The only discomfort was the irritation set up by the foley at the tip of the meatus. I found it uncomfortable to move about in bed or to walk to the bathroom because even slight movement of this foley caused discomfort. I circumvented this with my own Tylenol.

On the second, post-operative day that foley was finally removed and what a relief it was. Now I had to await the dramatic moment to discover whether or not I had sphincter control, whether or not I could start and stop my urinary stream at will.

I began to drink glass after glass of water in order to fill my bladder with urine for the big test. It felt good to get out of bed and walk around the room. While waiting for my bladder to fill I went for an exploratory walk up the hall, visiting others who were awaiting their turn at the cysto-scope.

Soon the urge to urinate came upon me.

I was instructed to save all urinary output until further notice so that the surgeon could determine whether post-operative bleeding was or was not excessive. I closed the bathroom door. There was a quart sized plastic urine collection bottle shaped like a water pitcher which I was instructed to "pee" in instead of the toilet. I held the pitcher under me. I released my sphincter and what a beautiful sight ensued. My urinary stream was at least one quarter inch in diameter. The urine rushed out of me at such a turbulent rate that I thought I was 18 years old again. There was no bleeding and no pain. There was no retention of urine and complete emp-tying of the bladder. And best of all, I had total control which some patients after this operation suffer for indefinite periods of time. I was so elated I could have demonstrated my prowess in the May Company's main window.

I remained in the hospital for five more days since I had to be observed for possible post-operative hemorrhage. But none has occurred since the operation.

I have made a complete recovery and I have never felt better in my life.

CHAPTER VIII

A JOURNEY DOWN THE BAJA

Although not an exotic place to visit, a solo journey down the center of Mexico's Baja or Lower California from Tijuana in the north to Cabo St. Lucas at its lowermost tip was the type of trip one should reserve for his retirement days. When the age of retirement arrives the possibility of losing one's life to Mexican highway bandits is not so serious as it is when one's children are still young and dependent.

It all started when I boarded a train in Baltimore for Chicago via Washington, D.C. In Washington I boarded the Capital Limited for an overnight trip to Chicago. I occupied a roomette which converted to a sleeper at bedtime.

Meals on the Amtrak are frozen, concocted in some catering establishment as on an airliner, and served directly from a microwave oven. Cutlery is not of the old "Pullman" vintage with white linen and pewter silver service. Today it's all disposable plastic. The train rattled and rolled and jerked and shook incessantly across West Virginia. Passing Pittsburgh, Canton, Ohio, Indiana and finally the densely industrial outskirts of Gary and Hammond, Indiana I arrived at Chicago's Union Station at 10 A.M. the next morning, after a sleepless night.

February in Chicago was cold and wintry. Walking the Loop, as I did in 1933 at the chicago World's Fair, was a frigid ordeal. After a six-hour layover, till 4 P.M., I boarded America's most luxurious and famous train, the old Santa Fe Chief now known as the Southwest Limited. It is operated by Amtrak, the government-subsidized passenger train system.

During the depression of 1937 I travelled by train across the United States, sat up in a coach and slept in the same seat for four nights en route to Los Angeles. I was 18 then. I worked on the Los Angeles Examiner, went to school at the University of Southern California, and used to eat breakfast at Clifton's Cafeteria for 18 cents. I vowed that some day, when I could afford it, I would check in at the Biltmore Hotel, like the affluent of that era, and relive a youthful fantasy.

Today at 66 and being partially retired, I occupied an entire room on that train, with 2 double beds, a shower, toilet, lounge chair, large picture window, personalized air conditioning and piped in music. I thought I would be able to enjoy a peaceful night's sleep as this luxurious train departed Chicago and headed west. Galesburg, Illinois, was the last city I saw before night fell. Then I went to the dining room and to my complete disappointment there was the same Amtrak frozen menu as on the Capital Limited. It was not worth eating. I had peanuts and coke for supper. I read till 10 P.M., then had the porter prepare one of my beds for sleep. Sleep was impossible. The train was excellent but the tracks were irregular, causing the train to sway from side to side, rattle and vibrate, especially after reaching speeds of 55 to 60 miles per hour. This type of swaying one might surmise would enhance sleep. But swaying wasn't its only fault. The rattling, vibration, jostling, shaking was as bad as the other train. It was once again impossible to sleep. In anticipation of the problem I took a sleeping pill. This also did not work. Fortunately, I only had one night to sleep on this train as it sped through Missouri and Kansas. I saw daybreak in Cimarron, Kansas, then I had tea in the dining room as we passed through Dodge City, and walked the passenger platform during a ten-minute stop in La Junta, Colorado. At 4 P.M. I left the train in Albuquerque, New Mexico, rented a Hertz car at the station and headed for a good night's sleep at a Holiday Inn.

The next day I drove from Albuquerque to Flagstaff and then to the Grand Canyon where I remained for the night and the following day. I acquired an individual cabin overlooking the Canyon.

Sunday I drove to Las Vegas via Kingman and the Boulder Dam. They still call it the Hoover Dam, but neither Herbert Hoover nor J. Edgard Hoover deserve this honor. The next day I drove to Death Valley then to Los Angeles where I bedded down at the Biltmore Hotel and ate at Clifton's Cafeteria on Broadway at 7th.

I drove to San Diego, left my car at the airport, then to Tijuana via taxi where I rented a Hertz Volkswagon for the long trip down the BAJA. No one at the border asked to see my passport. It seemed to me that anyone could enter Mexico at will.

BAJA, CALIFORNIA

The last time I was in Tijuana was in 1937 when it was a dirty, sleepy, sleezy village only several blocks long. Today, 43 years later, it is an enormous city, so large I had difficulty finding my way to its one major highway south known as Mexico Route 1, the 1059 mile road that runs the entire length of the Baja.

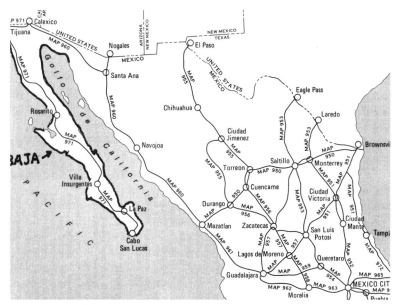

Map of Baja, Mexico, also know as Lower California

Baja means "lower" and the full name is Baja (pronounced "Baha") California. Although called "lower" California it is part of Mexico and is actually the upper part of the peninsula that broke off of Mexico a million years ago. In doing so, the Pacific Ocean rushed in and we now call that the Gulf of California. The Gulf waters border the east side of the 1000-mile Baja, the Pacific Ocean borders the west side. It is about 50 to 75 miles wide. The watery Gulf is about 100 miles across.

Before undertaking this voyage I was warned that numerous dangers lurked en route such as Mexican bandits, who, dressed as soldiers, would stop your car, rob you, then kill you and dispose of your car, your body, and you would just disappear from the face of the earth. The other dangers involved inadequate sleeping facilities where you would be attacked by bugs, mites, scorpions, and while asleep your car would be stolen or burglarized. I was told that gasoline was not available; that if my car broke down, there would be no transportation out of this Mexican wilderness; that so few people lived in the Baja that one could be lost forever; that there were neither hospitals or physicians should one become ill or meet with an accident.

What worried me most was the possible encounter with Mexican bandits because of the increased rate of unemployment and extreme hardship in

Mexico. Information from the AAA was also not very encouraging. My hopes ran slightly higher when I rented a Hertz car in Tijuana, Mexico, and they assured me that if any bandits lurked in the Baja hills, they would never attack a Hertz car and if this danger existed, Hertz would not permit their cars to travel the Baja. I was ready to cling to any assurance of safety and the yellow and black Hertz insignia on my red volkswagon became my mezuza of protection.

After almost an hour trying to find my way out of the intricate maze of unmarked streets and dusty unpaved side streets lined with every type of business, shop and enterprise imaginable, and asking at least half a dozen Mexicans for Autoroute Uno (one), I finally found Route 1 that led to the first major town south of Tijuana known as Ensenada, 68 miles down the Baja. So far the road was excellent and no sign of bandits. The biggest surprise was the toll booths. This 68-mile road to Ensenada was a limited access toll road. Many Californians ride down to Ensenada for fishing, resorting and horse racing so the toll road gives the impression that travelling in Mexico is as safe as in San Diego. I did not stop in this city of 150,000 Mexicans. I drove on through to the next town known as San Quintin which was 120 miles deeper into the Baja. It was now 5 p.m. and I was not about to drive this shoulderless, narrow two-lane highway at night. I checked in at the El Presidente Hotel in this tiny city whose name is reminiscent of the prison in California.

Hotel rooms in Mexico are superspacious but usually without telephones and without adequate wattage in their electric bulbs. I carry my own 200 watt bulbs and extension cords which I use to light up my room as I travel. I also have several gallons of U.S. spring water, an electric hotplate and an aluminum, 7-cup coffee pot since anyone who drinks Mexican water is as good as almost dead. This hotel bordered an extensive Pacific ocean beach and I spent the evening walking the beach and reading. The evening descended peacefully and an unusual silver sunset enveloped the sky over the Pacific.

I left San Quentin with a tank full of gas, thinking that so far everything was running smoothly. I arrived in the town of El Rosario and drove into the only PEMEX gas station in town since my gas tank was becoming anemic. There was no gas. They hadn't had gasoline for days and did not know when they would get any. This suddenly became the first ominous predicted problem to rear its head regarding travelling in the Baja. Would the Mexican bandits be next?

I drove on to the next village 76 miles down the road through beautiful, desert country thick with cactus; mountains and no people. The village was Catavina. I went into the PEMEX station. PEMEX is the only gas station and the only gas in Mexico since it is run and owned by the Federal Government. Once again, there was no gas. Now I was really worried. There was not only no gas, but practically no cars on the narrow, two-lane highway. If I became stuck here I frankly didn't know what I'd do. I mentally resolved to write a letter to the President of Mexico and give him hell about such an inhospitable, selfish situation especially since Mexico is trying to encourage tourists. The next town was Rosarito.

This was a further 65 miles away and my gas tank was really low. Fortunately the Volkeswagon gets excellent mileage per gallon. The scenery through this area was really outstanding but I could not enjoy a moment of it since my eye was constantly on my gas-tank gauge. The road began to go up hill towards a 2700 foot mountain summit. This required 2nd-gear driving which meant twice the gas consumption. Then down the mountain and into a vast dessert—the central desert of the Baja (where I absolutely did not want to be stranded). The variety of cactus here was unbelievable. Some were 25 feet tall. There were many cacti, some known as cardon cactus, cholla cactus, cirios cactus, yucca valida and elephant trees.

I came to a village. The gas station was closed. A sign on the pump said No Gas. I saw a man in a truck who had stopped to sell vegetables to some women. I offered him anything for gas. He said to go down the road one kilometer, turn left and there would be a small airfield. They might sell you some aviation fuel, but it's very expensive. Who cared about the expense! I dashed down the road, turned left and saw nothing. I kept going into the desert and sure enough there was a tiny landing strip for small planes, but no planes in sight. I drove up to a one-story house with a thatched roof, honked, and a young chap appeared. I needed "gasolina". He could spare five gallons which he had siphoned through a piece of garden hose from a five-gallon paint-thinner can. This very expensive gas cost less than gas does at Exxon stations in Baltimore. He saved the day.

The next big town was Guerrero Negro 80-miles down the road and finally, there was a station that had gas. This town is on the Pacific Ocean which can be seen from the highway as it is approached. It is famous as a breeding ground for whales which come down each February from the Artic to breed. I was so happy to get gasoline I forgot about the whales.

Baja California is known at the State of Baja California until you come to Guerrero Negro which is located on the 28th parallel. This divides Baja California, into two parts: the upper is the state of Baja California Norte, the lower part if called Baja California Sur. The license plates in this southern part of Baja are marked "B.C.S. Mexico". The "S" stands for Sur which means South. To demarcate this north-south division of the Baja, an enormous steel structure, supposed to be a monument, loomed up in the distance as if it were a tall draw bridge and I had to reduce my driving speed as I approached it. On closer examination I perceived it was one of those *avant garde,* ridiculous monuments, the brain child of a drug-ridden architect who designed it in a frenzy of a cocaine sniff. Perched on top of this monstrosity was the nest of the a pair of osprey's, tending their young.

Guerrero Negro is a large town located in the midst of a vast desert known as Vizcaino Desert. Five thousand people live here and produce salt by feeding sea water into 4-foot deep ponds. The desert sun causes rapid evaporation leaving a pure, hard salt. This is shipped to the U.S., Japan and Canada. With a happy heart made happier by a full gas tank I drove another 89 miles to the town where I spent the night. San Ignacio.

Many of these Mexican towns are named after Catholic saints. San stands for Saint and in this instance, Saint Ignatius. The Jesuits founded a mission here in 1728 and planted a few date palms. Now the place is so full of date palms that dates are exported as their chief crop along with figs, oranges and grapes. This town is in a deep valley called Arroyo surrounded by cactus-covered mountains. The streets are not paved; they are all dirt and dusty with chickens, roosters and cats and dogs running free, but each thatch-roofed hut has a G.E. electric meter.

This drive through the Baja is never without sight of the enormous cactus plants also known as cardon cactus. The climate and low rainfall are constant throughout the peninsula. The reason for the existence of the town of San Ignacio is the discovery of an underground river which emerges at the earth's surface and is the source of water for these otherwise impossible-to-exist date palms.

Each of the larger towns in the Baja has a hotel known as the El Presidente. These are all owned by the El Presidente chain of hotels and to look at the outside structure is to see an architect's dream. Large open gardens in the midst of the hotels, massive lobbies with wood and granite carvings, like nothing I've ever seen in the U.S. They have just exquisite lines and colored pastel stucco. But the rooms! The place where you sleep! The reason *d'etre* for the hotel is total stupidity. There are no telephones in the rooms. Air conditioning and heating systems never work. The sinks are too high off the floor. The spigots are corroded and difficult to adjust; there are no receptacles in the walls; lighting in the rooms is totally inadequate; the view from windows are obstructed by

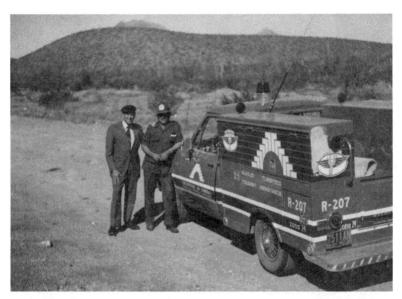

The "Green Angeles" are emergency service trucks operated by the Mexican Government in the Baja to assist stranded travellers with gas, flat tires, and mechanical failures.

dense over growth of palms, poinsettias and cactus. Hot water is seldomly available. And these are called the first-class hotels. The food in the hotel restaurants is actually dangerous to eat. Flies, ants and other bugs are everywhere since this is the tropics and it's difficult to keep these pests under control.

Until 1973, you could not travel down the Baja because there were no roads. But in 1973, Mexico completed the paving of this 1000-mile road, Route 1, known as the Transpeninsular Highway from Tijuana to the tip at Cabo San Lucas. There is a microwave telephone system connecting these towns, if you can find a telephone.

There is one organization operating in the Baja that is a real credit to Mexico. It is known as the *Green Angels,* and that's what they are. It is a government-operated fleet of green (usually a Dodge) trucks whose sole purpose is to provide *free* highway emergency service to tourists. They are manned by mechanics, some speak English, as well as Spanish, and carry spare auto parts, gasoline (at cost-no overcharge) and can summon assistance by radio.

I had heard of these angels and the first one I saw was a bright green truck parked by the roadside but with no driver. I parked my car to photograph the green truck and saw the driver urinating behind a cactus tree. Of course, I interviewed him and told him that he was truly a Mexican angel. They supposedly pass any given point on the Baja highway at least twice a day although I saw none driving during my day of gaslessness. The sight of this truck and the driver made me feel that driving the Baja was a lot safer than some of our remote areas in the U.S.

In the late 1800's, Baja became the forgotten peninsula as far as the government in Mexico City was concerned and it became a haven for criminals, smugglers and soldiers of fortune. Prohibition in the U.S., before Roosevelt, brought uncertain prosperity to the border towns between Mexico and the U.S., like Tijuana, where droves of Americans crossed the border, seeking booze and other more liberal pleasures. But in 1938, President Cardenas of Mexico routed out the bootleggers and gamblers and instituted intense agrarian and educational reforms. In 1952, the upper part of the Baja became Mexico's 29th state and in 1974 the lower half became the 30th state, the capital being the City of La Paz.

The next day with plenty of *gasolina* and the security of the Green Angels lurking somewhere along the highways, I drove through high mountains similar to those in California and arrived at the Gulf coastal town of Santa Rosalia. This was my first view of the Gulf of California. It looked like the Pacific Ocean but I saw it out of my left auto window on the east as I headed south instead of the actual Pacific Ocean which I had been seeing out of the right window to the west.

Santa Rosalia was quite a bustling town. There was one paved street with numerous shops and even a post office. The population is over 12,000 and earns its living mainly in the copper mines. What interested me especially about this town was a prefabricated church that sits in the town's main square. The church is made of prefabricated steel squares, bolted together, and trusses, arching across the ceiling also made of steel plates. What's so interesting about this? This church was designed by A. G. Eiffel in Paris, the designer of the Eiffel Tower, who designed it along with the Eiffel Tower for the 1898 World's Fair in Paris. The church was disassembled and shipped around Cape Horn to Santa Rosalia and it is used daily as a church here. I took interior and exterior pictures of this unusual structure.

Thirty-eight miles down the highway, I came to the town of Mulege where there was plenty of gas, dates, figs, bananas and olives. Soon one town became like another during this long drive through country that resembled in so many respects part of Arizona, Nevada and California.

From Mulege I went to Loreto where the first permanent settlement in California was made in 1697 by the Jesuits. Then to Ciudad Constitucion

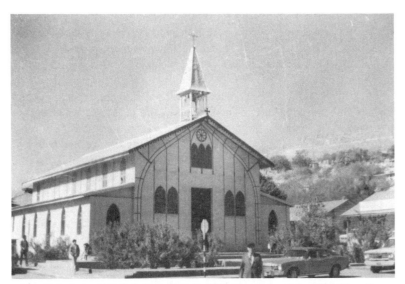

The all steel church built in Paris by A. G. Eiffel who designed the Eiffel Tower. It was disassembled, shipped to Santa Rosalia, Mexico, and reassembled there mainly with nuts and bolts.

where I spent the night in the town's top hotel which to my standards was a minus 5 star. It is known as the Mirabel, but the wall paper was peeling from the walls; the shower stall was slimy; but surprise, the water was hot. The largest bulb in the room was 40 watts. They grow cotton in the vicinity watered by deep wells since rain water all through the Baja is a rarity. This town also had the first traffic lights south of Ensenada.

The next big town prior to reaching the end of the line was 134 miles south to La Paz, but the road cuts across the Baja from west to east, on the gulf Coast. La Paz is the capital of Baja California Sur. During the summer it is very hot here but there is always a welcome breeze known as the Coromuel which is also the name of the ferry boat which runs between Cabo San Lucas and Puerto Vallarta.

On the last leg of the journey on Mexico's Route 1 I encountered towns such as El Triunfo, San Antonio, San Bartolo, Los Barriles, Buena Vista, Santiago, Miraflores, Santa Anita, San Jose Viejo, San Jose del Cabo and finally the grand entrance to the destination city at land's end which was Cabo San Lucas from which the ferry boat departs for Puerto Vallarta. The ferry trip involves 18 hours and 320 miles across the Pacific to the Mexican mainland.

The town of Cabo San Lucas at the southern tip of the Baja is a seaport town replete with luxury hotels, beaches and two Hertz depots. Boats dock in a U-shaped bay which in the 16th and 17th centuries was a favorite hiding place for pirates who lay in wait for Spanish treasure ships. Today it is packed with sailboats, fishing boats and luxury yachts, mostly flying the American flag.

I registered at the Hacienda Hotel which was also the deposition point for my Volkeswagon "bug". The *Coromuel,* the ferry boat which was to transport me to Puerto Vallarta was a large ocean-going vessel. I booked a luxury suite which included a bedroom, a sitting room, private bath and shower and was high up on the uppermost deck. The clerk at the government-operated ferry building advised me that that accommodation was most expensive and wouldn't I prefer a room with 5 other occupants. I assured her I could afford the luxury accommodation, thinking that a single hotel room at the Los Angeles Biltmore was over $100 and this couldn't be over $200 considering the transportation cost. The bill came to $35, and no tax! I smiled as I queried the clerk as to the accuracy of the price. She showed me the price list. To sit for the overnight sailing on a plastic chair, 10 abreast for 18 hours costs only 400 pesos which is less than $2 in U.S. currency. U.S. dollars are obviously quite valued in Mexico at this time.

This trip from Tijuana to Cabo San Lucas required four days of driving and three nights of sleeping. There was very little traffic on Mexico Route 1, the only road through the Baja. The essentials on this trip were the following: five gallons of mineral water purchased and bottled in the U.S., a seven cup metal coffee pot, a 110-volt cooking element (which resembles a burner from an electric stove) a 200-watt bulb, a 15-foot extension cord, a double socket, a jar of postum or instant coffee, a large drinking cup, a can opener, a sharp knife for cutting bread or onions, a bottle of paragoric, a wash rag, and a 5-day supply of tetracycline. These are the essentials.

The scenery was spectacular and inspiring and this was especially so because of the total abscence of billboard advertising, Dairy Queen ice cream stands, and other indications of our declining civilization. I had the feeling that this highway was cut through a tropical desert jungle where cactus in infinite variety propagated itself from the United States border all the way to Cabo San Lucas. The sky was uncontaminated by smog, and day after day the azure of Jerusalem's blue sky was always there for the looking. High mountains in the distance, or winding through hairpin turns while in them, afforded a kalidoscopic experience not unlike watching a kodachrome-slide show of unspeakable beauty. All of this accompanied by taped music such as Granada, Adios, and They've Got An Awful Lot of Coffee in Brazil.

At the harbor in Cabo San Lucas pelicans rested on row boats or on the sides of dinghies attached to fishing yachts. It was intriguing to see them dip their long bills into bait buckets and steal all the bait to the consternation of the fishermen. The harbor was thick with sea gulls and frigate birds. There was the occasional osprey and many of the wading shore birds, all running around poking their beaks in the sand. The frigates follow the sea gulls and when the sea gull snatched a fish from the Pacific, the frigate, in turn, snatched the fish from the sea gull's beak. Maintaining life is an eternal struggle for these free-soaring phantoms.

PUERTO VALLARTA

Puerto Vallarta is a hide-away winter resort for wealthy Americans and Canadians who are catered to by poverty-level Mexicans who live in shacks and one-room hovels. There is a shallow river that runs through the city and lining its banks are the tin shacks, and thatch-roofed huts of the Mexican working class. They wash their clothes in the river, rubbing the clothes and socks and shirts with soap against large boulders that form the banks of the river. They take their baths in the river, urinate in the river, brush their teeth in the river accompanied by their dogs who also cool off in its waters. The young Mexican girls emerge from their one-room shacks and walk to their work as cashiers in a bakery or grocery store, their neat jeans and spotless blouses, their artistic makeup and their *avant garde* stylish clothes and the elan with which they wear them seem to belie their humble abodes.

There are butcher shops for Canadians and Americans who buy imported meats thick with marbled fat at inflated prices. And other shops for Mexicans where fat in the meat of both pig and cow is visibly absent because the locally-grown animals eat only grass and no corn. The lean meat the Mexicans buy is usually pork. Their bread is tortillas and the lines of housewives form early in the morning in front of the tortilla shops. The streets in Puerto Vallarta are largely cobble-stoned and at many corners are fast food carts which specialize in different foods. A particularly popular food is roasted minced pork, chopped up fine which might include the skin of the pig along with its kidneys, heart, liver, muscle, tongue and eyes, all sauteed with onions and topped with a hot tomato and bean sauce and wrapped in a tortilla. This concoction is eaten for breakfast right out on the street and costs 20 cents. People stand in long lines to buy this and some of the vendors make as much as 300 to 500 dollars a day. Other vendors sell tortillas containing chopped-up beef and onions and others specialize in chopped-up shrimp and onions and hot peppers. I saw some of the pig meat cooking in preparation for the next morning's breakfast. It is cooked in water in a huge washtub outside a one room house, on a dirty road with no lid. The flies were most interested but a dog who came to sniff seemed repulsed.

Dust from unpaved streets contaminates the air, traffic is loud with horns and is bumper-to-bumper and a parking ticket (fine) costs 75 cents. First class hotels cost foreigners from $100 a day and up and that does not include food. The Pacific waters which wash the beaches of these innumerable hotels is largely contaminated by untreated sewage, so guests find refuge from the heat in chlorinated swimming pools approximate to the ocean. They are lucky they did not see all of the yellow and black sea snakes swimming in the bay. I saw these snakes every several hundred yards as the ferry entered the approach to Puerto Vallarta.

Kitchen industries abound in Puerto Vallarta. Concrete sewer pipes as well as bathroom tiles are manufactured by manual labor in back yards. Intricately-designed metal fences and railings are welded and constructed in small shops on any street, as is furniture, baskets, brooms, stained glass, pottery, etc. Even the roofs are not wasted space. I was pleased to see the dog who sleeps on the roof of the house below my apartment still there this year, along with his friend the cat and a rooster of magnificent voice.

The three days in Puerto Vallarta dawned and dusked in rapid succession and the time for flying back to Baltimore finally arrived. I presented my air ticket at the American Airline counter plus my Mexican entrance permit which was issued by my Baltimore travel agent. "Your entrance permit was not stamped with the date you entered Mexico" said the agent. I explained that I entered Mexico by taxi, went to the Hertz Drive-It-yourself agency in Tijuana, drove the Baja and came to Puerto Vallarta by ferry boat. He was so sorry but without an entrance stamp he could not accept my already-paid-for ticket. I would have to go to the immigration office at the farther end of the airport. Meanwhile, he would hold my baggage at his desk.

It was hot and sweaty at the airport and I had visions of my niece who was once detained for 5 days in Mexico City with a similar immigration infraction. I entered the door with the word *migracion* inscribed over it. It was a bare room with an old desk, an oak chair, and a tired immigration official sitting there waiting to hear a tale of woe he has apparently heard many times before. *"Buenos Tardes"* (good afternoon) he said. It was Sunday, February 17, 1985, one hour before departure for Dallas, Texas and Baltimore. I showed him my airline ticket and my entrance permit. "When did you enter Mexico?". I told him Friday, February 8th and repeated the story, adding that at Tijuana no one had asked to see any papers, in fact no official sees anyone entering Mexico at all, you just drive through. "Your word means nothing. You are illegally in Mexico according to this paper. You could have been here for years. Also, it says here you entered by auto, you checked this yourself. To whom did you sell your car?"

I was infuriated. I said, *"Un momento por favor"*. I explained more of my wonderful experience down the Baja and showed him my Hertz Rental Car receipt which showed the date I rented the car and turned it in. "But this Hertz receipt is not an official entrance stamp into Mexico. Anyone can present such a receipt. I am sorry but I cannot permit you to leave Mexico until the head of *Migracion* hears your case and since today is a holiday, Sunday, your case cannot be heard till tomorrow at number 600 Morales St., 1st floor in Puerto Vallarta," he stated firmly.

"But my flight leaves in an hour and I must get back to Baltimore!" I contended. Even my Johns Hopkins card didn't help. "Senor, you can go to jail for this. I am sorry but I have no authority to stamp your certificate. It is a legal offense. Good day!" he responded. I was irritated, infuriated, exasperated, frustrated, and helpless. I went back to the American Airline Desk, told the agent of my dilemma. He said I'll change your reservation to Monday. He assured me that if he gave me a boarding card without the stamped immigration certificate (which he couldn't do in the first place) they would not let me board the plane and we could both go to jail!

What to do? My brother who lives in Puerto Vallarta part of the year made a phone call to Mario, his agent for emergency "pull" situations. Mario's phone did not answer. Buzzy meanwhile had gone to see the head of the airport migracion officaldom, a man who knows Buzzy personally, who has been entertained at his house and who saw me disembark from the ferry. He could do nothing.

We were standing now in the middle of the crowded hustle and bustle of the airport trying to decide where to spend the night and talking of the possibility of a similar intransigent situation on the morrow in the *migracion* office and wondering if I would ever get out of Mexico without driving back up the Baja to Tijuana and having them stamp my certificate as if I had just entered this neighboring country.

All of a sudden, as if by Providence, Mario walked up to my brother Buzzy greeting him with a merry hello. Buzzy could not believe his eyes. It was like the Israeli victory over the Egyptians in the Six-Day War—a miracle. He told Mario (who has all kinds of not only local connections but federal connections as well and is a millionaire land and hotel owner) that his brother here needs a *"migracion"* certificate.

Without another word of explanation Mario took the certificate and my Hertz receipt, disappeared for 10 minutes while we waited in the middle of the airport. He returned with a little white piece of paper, with a stamp on it and official signature and refused any compensation.

It was a miracle that happened under circumstances that seemed so natural, like the victories of the Israelis over their enemies in the three Israeli wars. Is there Providence operating in history, in the lives of men? I am certain there is.

In the meantime, the seat I had reserved was sold to another passenger and the plane was fully booked—except for first class. So I travelled first class back to Baltimore, on a coach class ticket—a little justice from American Airlines.

CHAPTER IX

A DRIVE ACROSS
THE UNITED STATES

White contemplating retirement, I decided to attend an anesthesia convention in Loma Linda, California, by driving across the United States, starting from Baltimore.

I followed route I-81 which winds through the Shenandoah Valley, bordered on both sides, about 20 miles apart, by the never-ending Appalachian range of mountains. This mountain range is to the East coast of the U.S. what the Rocky Mountain range is to the West coast. If there were no road markers to announce the crossing from Maryland into Virginia, West Virginia and Tennessee I would be unable to differentiate the states. The spring season had transformed the roadside into blazes of yellow forsythia, purple cherry blossoms and that beautiful light green of newly-born leaves, interspersed with white dogwood blossoms. All four states exhibit the same degree of spring blossoming.

I stopped in Knoxville to visit the grave of my grandfather, Saul Friedmond. This is the spelling on the grave stone. I have never met this gentleman, but since he lived here and became the principal of a Hebrew school, I found myself gazing at old, old buildings and thought surely he must have seen these buildings too. It's like gazing upon a 300-year-old oak tree at George Washington's birthplace and realizing that George also saw that tree. The tree and buildings seem to bind the past to present reality.

I established contact with a man who knew of my grandfather who arrived in Knoxville in 1912 and lived here until his death in 1918. The man is Jacob Corkland who was one of my grandfather's students. This Mr. Corkland, aged 79, is head of a real estate firm, and was very fond of my grandfather. Mr. Corkland sat behind his desk and slowly unveiled the years of long ago when he was 10 years old, and attended my grandfather's Hebrew school. He spoke of him with love and tenderness and had tears in his eyes as memories flashed back.

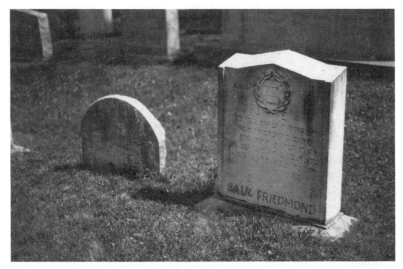

The grave of my grandfather, Saul Friedmond who was buried in Knoxville, Tennessee.

He came to Knoxville from Baltimore because a Baltimore Cantor who used to come to Knoxville to lead services on Rosh Hashanah and Yom Kippur told him they needed a learned man to head a Hebrew school in the Knoxville community.

Corkland said he was a brilliant man, very religious, and would not eat in anyone's home. He did his own cooking in the small apartment where he lived close to the Shul.

My grandfather took an especial interest in Jacob Corkland and taught him to read, not only his own Maftir for his own Bar Mitzvah, but all the weekly Maftirs. To this day Corkland is called on to read the Maftir of the week when there's no Bar Mitzvah, since he is the only one who can do it without preparation.

He told me of my grandfather's library. He was studying, and he wrote many commentaries in the German language from which he read to Corkland. Corkland said that his personal orthodox orientation to this very day is due totally to my grandfather's influence.

I was then taken to the graveyard and I photographed his gravestone. He is buried next to a marker under which are buried old prayer books and prayer shawls. His name on the tombstone is

SAUL FRIEDMOND

The cemetery is the only Jewish one in Knoxville. Half is maintained by the orthodox Jews and the other half, demarcated by the single driveway through the cemetery, is reserved for the reform Jews.

It took all day to cross Tennessee. It's the longest state in the nation, next to Texas, in an east-west direction. Indiana, Illinois and a part of Ohio can fit in its east to west extent. There were many hills and mountains in Tennessee since it sits in the midst of the Appalachian mountain range.

I spent a weekend in a motel in Memphis, Tennessee, right on the bank of the Mississippi River which I could see from my room. Across the wide Mississippi is Arkansas which was also visible from my window.

The sign reading "Arkansas Welcomes You" was suspended across the girders in the middle of the bridge which spans the wide, brown, swiftly-flowing Mississippi River. The river is the natural boundry between Tennessee and Arkansas. The sign is exactly at the midpoint of the river.

The state of Arkansas varies hardly at all from the landscape of parts of Maryland. Soy beans and cotton are the main crops, and much of the land is flat from horizon to horizon.

The remarkable thing about travel is the interstate marking of Federal highways by signs which read, for example, I-40, the one I'm following going West. The interstate highways are a marvel to behold. From coast to coast these ribbons of concrete flow ever onward without cross-roads and stop lights, and without the danger of a head-on collision since the opposite lane is separated by a 20 foot or more grass, divider strip. When I left Tennessee I set my cruise control at 55 miles an hour and if I had had an endless supply of gas and an unlimited bladder capacity I could have driven non-stop across the entire state of Arkansas and Oklahoma without even slowing down.

These superhighways that stretch from ocean to ocean and Canada to Mexico cost billions to construct, but I feel they are worth it. But wouldn't it be a travesty if these beautifully-engineered thruways remain unused because we run out of fuel?

Halfway across Oklahoma I beheld the first hint of the West, and its wide open spaces. Prior to Oklahoma I found it difficult to find any radical change from Maryland's landscape. But I saw the gradual change in the landscape as the trees became more scarce. The land became flat then rolling. Instead of farms there were ranches with grazing cattle and the unique kind of fences that keep cattle off the highways.

For several years I have been recording my favorite old songs from FM stations on to cassettes. I brought many of these cassettes with me.

With a pillow behind my head, the cruise control at 55, I renewed old memories conjured up by the songs such as Blue Moon, Willow Weep for Me, Stormy Weather, Love Walked Right In and Smoke Gets In Your Eyes. Anyone who does not take along a tape recorder on a solo trip like this, knows not how to live. I also have symphonies by Tchaikovsky, Ravel and Brahms for my "lighter" moments. The trip has been sheer joy and I have not lost sight of a single blade of grass along the route.

Clinton, Oklahoma, is a dot on the map, with the usual collection of gas stations, motels, a general store and wide, wide, typical western streets. It's an important stopping place because of the Holiday Inn.

Holiday Inns cost more, but they're worth it. The sinks and bathtubs are not partially stopped up. An old cigarette butt cannot be found hiding behind the bathroom door. The keys work in the doors and the bulbs are bright enough to read by. In addition, the sheets are soft and not starched and the beds are uniformly comfortable. I cannot say the same for Best Western, Hyatt Hotels, Travel Lodge, or lesser names.

Soon after leaving Clinton, Oklahoma, I crossed the border into Texas, into the part that protrudes up into the map called the "Pan Handle". It did not take long to cross this part of Texas. But it was certainly Texas. Soon there were almost no trees, just endless stretches of grasslands for grazing cattle that will appear later in McDonald's hamburgers. The roads were paved to perfection and so smooth that even a rough-riding Mercedes would feel like a Rolls Royce.

Soon I arrived in the true, true West. I crossed from Texas into New Mexico, right at the sign which said "Mountain Time Zone", which meant turning my watch back another hour.

New Mexico is much like Old Mexico as far as landscape is concerned. It has beautiful rock formations, tumbleweeds, and vast unpeopled spaces.

I deviated from Route 40 which is still part of the old Southern Route to California known as Route 66. I turned north and drove to Santa Fe, New Mexico, thinking I would find a little town several blocks long with a familiar old railroad station that I visited 44 years previously. What a surprise! The little two-block town is now several miles long in every direction, packed with people, streets, new homes, schools, motels and Tasty-Freeze ice cream. I had to ask directions to the Holiday Inn. There are 3 or 4 exits on the expressway which by-passes the city, so large has it grown. Nothing remained the same. At the Holiday Inn I couldn't even hear the Santa Fe train whistle which 44 years ago would have been one block off the main street.

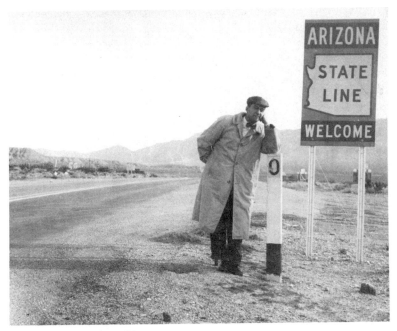

Entering Arizona from New Mexico.

I travelled from Santa Fe, New Mexico, and entered Arizona. First I entered Albuquerque, then passed through such towns as Holbrook, Winslow, Grants, Flagstaff, Gallup, then the Petrified Forest, Williams and on to the Grand Canyon.

The turn-off of I-40 or (U.S. 66) at the marker which says *The Grand Canyon, 62 Miles,* is a very nostalgic turn for me because it invariably turns me on! I have taken this turn off innumerable times, usually coming from California. The first time was in 1938, and the times in between I have lost count. I even have a song which I sing to myself as soon as I make this turn. The song is 44 years old and I still sing it. This time I had it on my tape recorder, having captured it from an FM station last year. The song is titled Two Sleepy People. I stopped my car briefly at the Grand Canyon sign and ran through the cassettes until I found the song. I played it over and over, interspersed with My Reverie during the 62 mile drive to the edge of the earth.

The 62-mile drive to the Canyon is a thrilling experience in itself. The road is at the 7000-foot elevation and traverses the Kaibab National For-

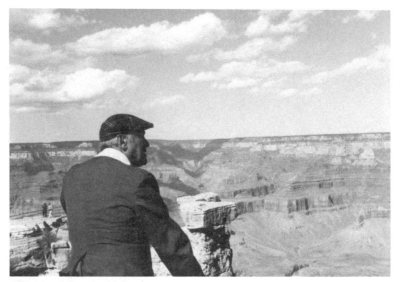

At the Grand Canyon.

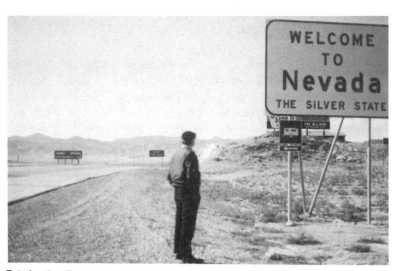

Entering the silver state—Nevada. This is also the start of the Pacific Time Zone.

est, a forest of unique design consisting of green needled fir, hemlock and spruce trees which live only at this high elevation. Pine cones are inches deep at the base of the trees and the rarefied air is pungent with the smell of evergreen. I did not drive this 62-mile stretch at the legal speed limit of 55 miles an hour. I set my speed control at 40 and in a Cadillac, it felt as if I were creeping along. At this slower speed I could revel in the beauty and shapes of the trees, and follow with my eyes an occasional wild deer or rabbit as it dashed across the highway. Since the Kaibab is a government preserve, no advertising signs or McDonald's hamburger signs pollute the scenery.

As the Grand Canyon draws nearer, the trees grow taller, and all of a sudden the Canyon appears. This great wide chasm permits a glimpse into the very depths and bowels of the earth. It is so vast, so deep, so enormous, so indescribable, and so awe-inspiring. And its appearance is never quite the same. It's like a sunset that always varies with ever-changing cloud formations. The canyon's color, its lights and shadows are in constant motion, especially when isolated puffs of clouds drift between the canyon and the sun.

As many times as I have revisited the Grand Canyon, each experience has produced a different mood, and a different spectacle. Whenever I see it I realize then and there that I will return again and again to revel in this wonder of the world.

It was snowing when I reached the canyon, and snow on the evergreens of the Kaibab and snow falling within the canyon is a sight that defies description. But it is also a mood. There's an elevation of one's spirit here, a thankfulness for eyesight, a mood that tells of man's fraility and man's inadequacy against the forces of nature. The Grand Canyon is a great force in instituting humility in man.

I ate supper in the El Tovar, the inn on the canyon's south rim that dates back to the turn of the century. It is still an elegant place. They even present you with a chilled fork in a folded napkin with which to eat your salad. This fork is over and above the regular fork setting. This is supposed to keep the salad cold when it is forked from the plate to your mouth. Heaven forbid that a room temperature fork at your place setting might raise the temperature of your cut-up lettuce by a tenth of a degree before your mouth warms it to body temperature. This is like cherries jubilee, the original restaurant fake. I don't go for that kind of public pretense, especially when the waiter presents it to you with slight bow and one hand behind his back. I showed him, I didn't even use his chilled fork!!

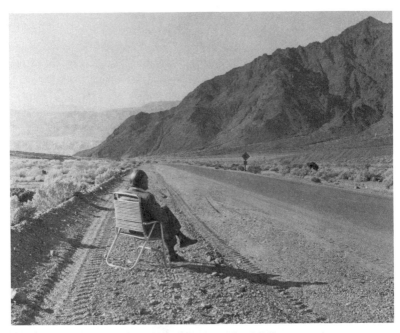

Reveling in the silence of the lifeless mountains of Death Valley.

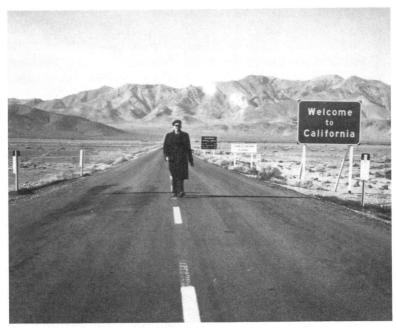

Entering California at the Nevada border.

I left the canyon at dawn, and drove via Cameron and the canyon's north rim region through another stretch of the Kaibab to Fredonia, Utah. This drive is one of the most scenic in the entire U.S. I went through Hurricane and St. George, Utah, and crossed the border into Nevada. I stopped for the night in Las Vegas, Nevada, at Tam O'Shanter Motel and saw the Shecky Green show at the Sands. The fish and vegetables were swimming in butter, and Shecky Green told the same Ka Ka jokes he told when I saw him five years previously.

The next day I drove from Las Vegas to Death Valley, sat for an hour on a folding chair, revelling in the silence of the surrounding mountains. Then I drove across the mountain range to the Wildrose exit from Death Valley into the Panamint Valley, with the Panamint Mountains to my left and the high Sierra Nevada range to my right, through Trona, Mojave, and into Palmdale and finally Los Angeles via the Hollywood Freeway.

About 30 miles outside of Las Vegas, Nevada there is a sign which is a sort of goal marker. It is a large sign, about the size of a home movie screen, and for anyone travelling from the east to California the sight of it is an important milestone. It sits out in the midst of the Nevada desert, a wasteland of sage brush and tumbleweeds and cactus. It sits there in the midst of utter silence except for the sound of the wind, which in May is thick with the scent of small yellow and orange desert blossoms. I stopped before this sign and turned the motor off so I could hear the silence of the desert, and stared at these beautiful words: *"Welcome to California"*. I stopped my car in Nevada so I could walk across the boundary line into C-A-L-I-F-O-R-N-I-A. I read the sign out loud several times so I could hear the melody of that far away dream since childhood—C-A-L-I-F-O-R-N-I-A. I had to repeat the word out loud so my ears could hear it, so my lips could form it, so that I could grasp every facet of this moment which has never ceased to thrill me. As many times as I have crossed borders into California, whether from Arizona or Nevada, or Mexico, I am still exhilarated by the magic of this wonderful state.

I drove very slowly for the first five miles into California so I could savour the reality of my fulfilled goal. How beautiful were the mountains, how vast the deserts, how silent and undisturbed was nature, and how at peace and content was I. I was so happy that the entrance into California was not like entering New York via a crowded bridge or through the suffocating odors of the Holland or Lincoln Tunnel, or through an over-crowded expressway.

I checked in at the Biltmore Hotel in Los Angeles at Fifth and Olive Streets and did several nostalgic things during the ensuing six days.

On one day I parked my car and with tape recorder I sat in Westlake Park. First I read the Examiner. Then I watched the pidgeons. I listened to the traffic, observed the palm trees, and watched parents run after playful children. I saw old, retired men walk slowly to a bench and carefully sit down, as older men will do.

Why did I sit in Westlake Park in the Chicano area of Los Angeles, about a mile from the inner city? Because 44 years ago, under pressure from the Examiner where I was working my way through the University of Southern California, I would sit in this park in order to hide from a roving Examiner executive who might find me goofing off. It was like the ditch digger on a WPA project who stops digging when the overseer's eyes are diverted.

I sat in the park thankful that I did not have to sell classified advertising and make that plague of a quota, and thought about my life. I tried to recapture the misery of those bygone days by playing taped music indigenous to that era. And when I could, for a fleeting moment, actually recapture the feeling and the mood, it was evanescent, brief, like a lightening flash, and then it was gone. I returned then, to the reality of the moment—to the reality of being not poverty stricken, not ever-fearful of losing the security of my Examiner job, but to the pleasant reality of being free of financial dependence, of having made something worthwhile of my life, of looking about me at the poor Chicanos, most of whom were unemployed, and being happy to have escaped from that emotional prison.

There's a peculiar reverse logic in this type of behavior. I go to great effort to recreate the unhappiness of an event that occurred 44 years ago and then reverse the unhappiness with today's reality. Fortunately many of the landmarks that I knew in my teens in Los Angeles are still there; the Examiner Building at Broadway and 11th, the first home I called on to sell an ad, on Rampart Boulevard and 3rd Street, the RKO Studio buildings on Gower Street, now a branch of Paramount Studios, the Griffith Park Observatory, and an old tree on Rosemont Avenue where I used to live. I even stopped in nostalgic reverie in front of an apartment house on Occidental Blvd. where every Friday afternoon I would sit on a stone bench in the lobby and read the latest issue of Life Magazine left there by the postman for the occupant who had not yet returned from work. To have bought the magazine for 10 cents was what breakfast cost and that was extravagant.

So powerful is this nostalgic phenomenon that I drove each morning from Hollywood to Clifton's Cafeteria on Broadway at 7th in downtown Los Angeles to eat breakfast in the cafeteria I used to eat in when I became more affluent and could afford to pay 35 cents for breakfast instead of 13 cents when I first arrived in Los Angeles in 1936. And I paid $2.00 to park my car so I could eat at Clifton's. Two dollars was the weekly cost of a room I lived in on Fifth Street 44 years ago while working at the Examiner and studying at the University of Southern California.

CHAPTER X

HOW I HAND BUILT A DREAM
HOUSE OF GLASS

When I was 31 years old I built a 10-room, ranch house in the Mt. Washington section of Baltimore with my own hands. My four children grew up there. All of them married, moved out to their own homes and produced 11 grandchildren.

This Mt. Washington house was surrounded by trees so dense that it was impossible to see a sunrise or a sunset.

I found a high hill of six acres in Frizzellburg, a section of Westminster, about 30 miles from Baltimore. I decided to build, with my own hands, a house of glass so that I could see the sunrise and sunset, unobstructed by trees or other houses.

I designed the house on paper, gave it to an architect who drew up the detailed blue prints, which are a requirement for a building permit in Carroll County.

The contract for purchase of this six-acre hill stipulated that if I drilled a well which produced no water, I would receive my deposit back. I employed a well digging company and at a depth of 800 feet water gushed out at the rate of 8 gallons a minute.

I bought the land and started construction in April, 1985.

Next I employed a man with a bulldozer. After staking out the outline of the house by placing stakes in the ground and attaching a cord line to the stakes, the bulldozer came in and scooped out an eight foot cellar. Obviously, I could not dig such a ditch by hand.

Next I employed a contractor who poured concrete, cellar walls and floors. In the dug-out cellar ditch he hand dug a six-inch deep trench 18 inches wide, lined it with reenforcing steel into which concrete was poured. This constituted the footing. When the footing concrete dried, steel forms 8 feet high were placed on the footings. These steel forms had an 8 inch space between them. Concrete was then poured in between these forms. The tops of the forms were levelled by a transit instrument since the top of the steel forms, once the concrete hardened and the steel forms

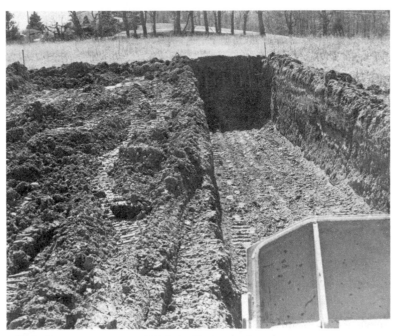

The bulldozer scoops out an eight foot cellar in one afternoon.

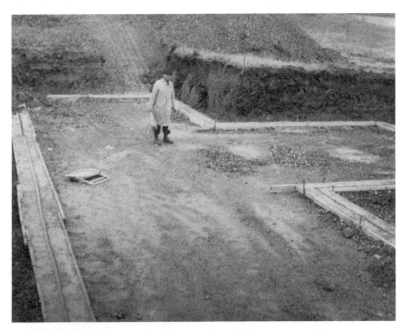

On the dirt floor of the dugout cellar, 2 × 6 wood forms are placed. Concrete is then poured into the forms to form the footing.

were removed, would constitute the cellar walls on which the house would rest.

Once the cellar contractor removed his steel forms and departed, the construction of the house from this point onward was totally in and by my own hands.

The next stop was laying a 2 inch layer of fiberglass insulation on top of the 8-inch concrete walls. On top of that I laid a wooden plate which consisted of 2 × 8 treated lumber. The plate was attached to the concrete foundation by strips of galvanized steel which had been embedded at 4 foot intervals in the top of the soft concrete before it hardened.

The next step was placing 2 × 12 joists across the top of the foundation and nailing them to the 8-inch plate.

Roof supports, consisting of 4 × 6 posts were placed on the plate at eight foot intervals. The floor was then nailed to the 2 × 12 joists. The floor consisted of 4 × 8 × 5/8 inch sheets of exterior plywood. Window outlets were attached to the upright roof supports.

With the floor nailed to the joists, I then had a solid surface on which to stand to construct the roof supports. This was done by nailing 2 × 2 × 10's across the tops of all the upright 4 × 6 posts.

The triangular roof trusses I had constructed at a lumber yard. The size and number of these trusses were determined and designed by a computer. These were delivered to the building site by a large truck.

These trusses were very heavy and I was unable to lift them into place myself. I hired three men to help me. These trusses were lifted and nailed into place on the 2 × 10's and with three men it was accomplished in one day.

The next day 4 × 8 × 1/2 inch exterior plywood was nailed to these trusses and the roof was finished except for the shingles which went on several days later. I could now work on the interior of the house protected from rain.

Meanwhile, I had a septic tank company dig out a large pit for the septic tank which they installed. Certain operations such as installing a two-ton septic tank cannot be managed without the help of heavy lifting equipment. So I had to have this done for me.

I then began the delineation of the rooms by constructing the walls of the rooms by laying 2 × 4's on the floor. I nailed the partition together on the floor then lifted the partition into place and nailed it to the plywood floor below and to the trusses above to which the ceiling would later be attached.

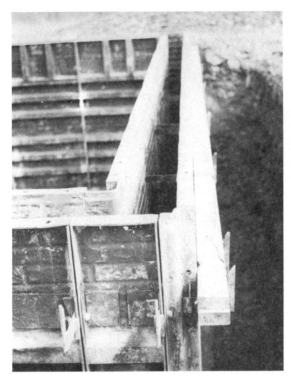

Steel forms 8 feet high and 8 inches between the forms, rest on the previously poured footings. Concrete is poured between the forms to form the cellar walls.

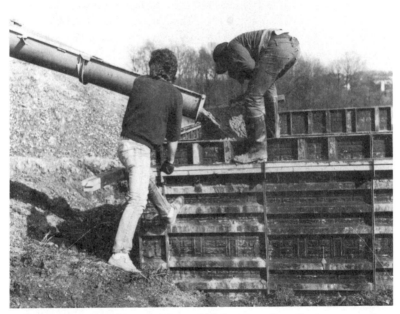

Concrete being poured into steel forms which form the cellar walls.

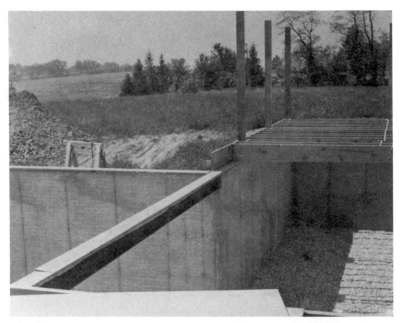

Steel forms removed showing concrete poured cellar walls, on top of which the 2 × 8 wooden plate is held in place by steel foundation strips which were previously imbedded in the concrete before it hardened. Also shown are the 2 × 12 joists and the 4 × 6 posts resting on the plate. The posts will support the roof.

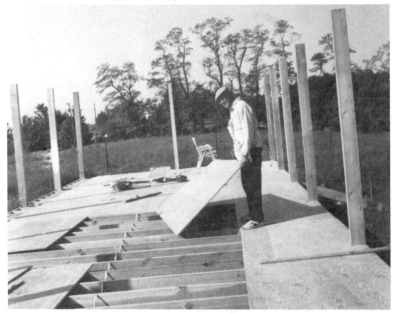

The subfloor consisted of 4 × 8 sheets of 1/2-inch plywood which were nailed to the underlying joists.

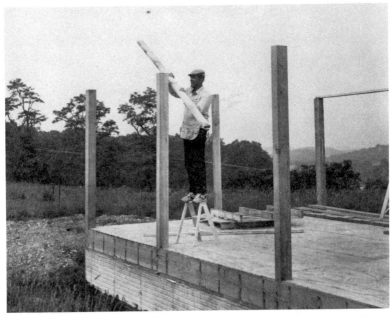

2 × 4's are placed across the upright posts as a platform to hold the larger 2 × 10's on which will be placed the trusses which support the roof.

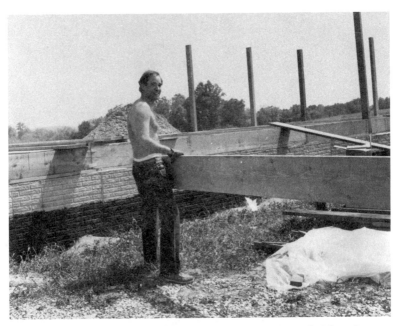

My son, Dr. Frank Shane, lends a helping hand on his day off from dental practice.

I purchased pre-hung doors which I fitted into the 2 × 4 partitions. At this point none of the windows or outside doors were in, and rain did find its way into the house making puddles on the plywood floors. Some rainwater leaked into the cellar forming puddles down there.

The next big step was the installation of the 5 × 8 foot double glazed windows. These giant windows could not be lifted by one man. The glass company that fabricated them for me also installed them in the metal frames which I had previously installed between the 4 × 6 posts that supported the roof.

Outside sliding glass doors I installed and with that the house could now be locked against theft.

The ceilings and inside walls were not yet in since the next big operation was installing the burglar alarm system and wiring the house. This I did myself. The kitchen wall where the sink was to be installed I roughed in receptacle boxes every 16 inches for the width of the kitchen which was 12 feet. All outside lights were on a low voltage relay system so that outside lights could be turned on or off from inside the house, at my bed and at the front door hallway.

The mailbox at the entrance to the one-block long driveway was fitted with a switch which was connected to an 18-volt bulb in the hallway of the house. When the mailman delivered mail, opening the box caused a buzzer to buzz and the 18-volt light remained lit telling me that the mail had been delivered.

The burglar system which I designed and installed had several interesting features. Should a door be forced or a window broken all the outside lights would go on, three sirens would blast off, and on the roof a strobe light flashed on and off every second.

I installed an infrared signal device between two posts that straddled the driveway. Should any person or automobile break the invisible beam, buzzers in every room and and all three bathrooms would buzz. This signal alerted me that someone was coming up the driveway. The beam was high enough off the ground so that it would not be broken by a dog or cat.

I built a flagstone platform in the living room on which I placed a modern wood burning stove. By opening the door of the stove it became an open fireplace. A routine fireplace in a private home is considered to be very inefficient since it draws heat out of the house and sends it up the chimney.

I installed at the point where my bed would be, a thick cable of wires which would serve to turn lights on and off in the room, outside the

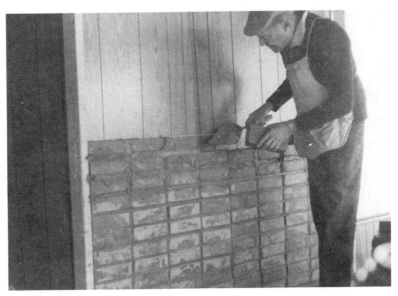

Constructing the brick fireplace wall.

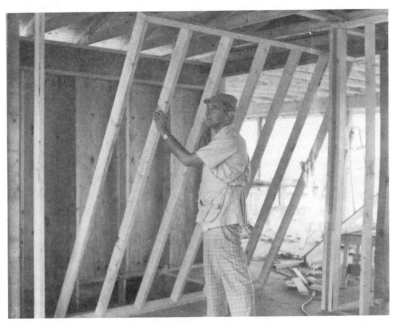

Interior walls are constructed by assembling 2 x 4's on the floor, then lifting them up into position.

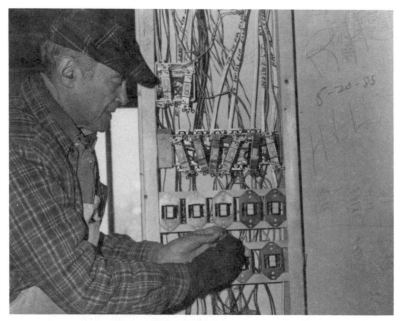

Installing the low and high voltage electric wiring.

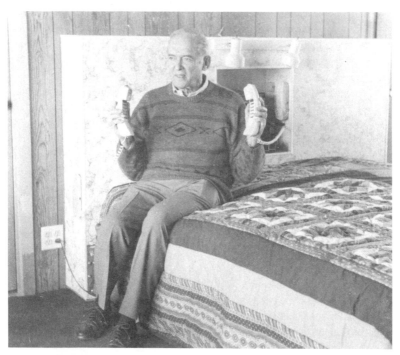

The headboard of the bed with phones on either side to facilitate answering without turning over.

house, operate a bell in the kitchen which tells whomever is in the kitchen that I need attention, operates a switch to turn on or off an overhead, electric fan should the bed become too warm in summer and for spreading the heat evenly in winter. Another set of wires was for the bedside telephone. Another set was for operating a cassette music system, and another set to rotate the outdoor TV antenna for better reception. All of this was designed so that I would not have to get out of bed to operate any of these switches.

I built a headboard for the bed which was as wide as two twin beds and high enough for me to sit up in bed and lean against when reading. In the center of the headboard was an opening 18 inches by 8 inches into which was placed the cassette music system, a telephone, the rotor mechanism for the TV aerial, and the heating controls for an electric blanket. Three low-voltage switches were attached to the side of this opening to operate the overhead fan, lights in the room, and all the outside lights should I hear noises in the night.

The headboard opening had one phone and the outside of the headboard another phone so that I could answer the phone while lying on my right side or the left side.

There are three bathrooms, two on the main floor and one in the cellar.

The main bath had a large jacuzzi instead of a bathtub plus a shower. There were two phones in this bathroom, one at the jacuzzi and one between the commode and the shower. There was also an overhead fan over the jacuzzi. The other two bathrooms had shower stalls only.

The heating system is a heat pump which provides cooling in summer through the same ducts. There are overhead fans in every room.

Once all of these wires were installed it was necessary to contact the Carroll County electrical inspection department for official approval. The inspector approved all the wiring except for one switch. This switch which operated the jacuzzi I had placed on the wall so that I could operate the jacuzzi motor while sitting in the jacuzzi. The electrical code was just changed, he explained, and required that a switch to operate a jacuzzi must be 5 feet away so that someone in the jacuzzi would be unable to touch the switch while sitting or standing in water. This was a safety precaution to prevent electrocution should the grounding circuitry become disconnected. Of course, I removed the switch and installed it five feet away in a most inconvenient location.

Now that the wiring was approved I could now begin applying paneling to the walls and ceilings. I did not start the paneling until the plumbing inspector approved all the copper pipes which would also be covered with the paneling.

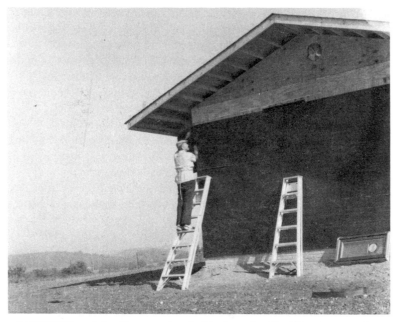

Asphalt impregnated roofing paper is nailed to plywood walls which acts as a moisture barrier. Vinyl siding will be applied over this.

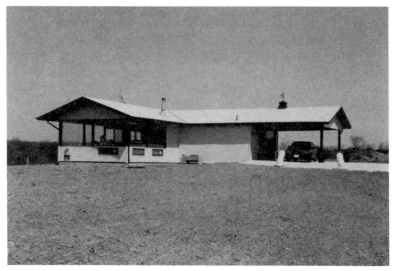

The finished house.

The panels were of oak plywood except one room which consisted of sheet rock which was later painted.

I then contacted an insulation contractor who blew the insulation into the roof to a height of 10 inches. I had previously installed paneling in the ceilings which supported the 10 inches of blown-in insulation.

I installed fiberglass bats between each 2 × 6 outside joists in those few outside walls where there was no glass.

The outside walls of the house consisted of plywood sheets 4 × 8 in size. On to this I hammered long sheets of asphalt-impregnated roofing paper which acted as a moisture barrier. Vinyl siding was then nailed to the roofing-papered surface of the exterior plywood covering.

In the cellar I installed a 16 millimeter motion picture arc lamp projector and a movie screen. Since the house was 62 feet long I could project an image almost as large as that seen in a theatre.

The final operation was the installation of wall to wall carpeting. My next door neighbor, being a carpet-laying expert, installed the carpeting. On July 2, 1986, I moved in after a year and three months of construction.

CHAPTER XI

THE INVESTIGATION

One day in 1956, while in the operating room at the Lutheran Hospital I received a phone call from a strange man who introduced himself as an agent of the Bureau of Internal Revenue. He requested in ever-so-polite a manner that I meet with him in the Federal Building for a routine check on my income tax returns going back over several years. I told him that I had never executed my own returns, and that my accountant was charged with sole authority, and wouldn't he prefer to speak with my accountant instead. He insisted that I appear personally but that my accountant could accompany me if I so desired.

Practically everyone whose income was in the five figure range was interviewed at one time or another by the income tax investigators so I considered this a mere routine request. Little did I realize the cauldron into which I was about to step.

At the appointed time my accountant and I visited the income tax investigator. My accountant had been preparing my annual returns for many years and I never questioned his judgment. He was not only a C.P.A. but a lawyer as well, and was considered, so I thought, an expert on tax law.

We sat on chairs in front of the investigator's desk, which was located in a small glass-enclosed cubby, one of many in a line of cubbies. The investigator, whom I shall call Lawson, was the Hollywood version of a detective. His face was tense and unhappy and it appeared as if a smile had never graced his gargoyle-like features.

I introduced my accountant to him and without so much as a how-do-you-do he launched into the business at hand.

"Dr. Shane," he began, his questions always directed at me and not at the accountant, "would you tell me how many rooms you have in your house?"

"Ten," I answered, wondering what this had to do with income tax.

"How many of these ten rooms do you use in the pursuit of your profession?"

"Just one, my study," I answered, still wondering what he was up to.

"If you are using only one room why then do you claim and deduct 50 percent of your household expenses on your income tax which would be the equivalent of using five rooms? You are obviously entitled to deduct only one-tenth, not one half of your expenses."

"Mr. Lawson," I fired back at him, "I know nothing about income tax laws and regulations. My accountant here who is an expert set up this deduction schedule years ago and I have no reason to question his judgment. I suggest you ask him."

A verbal hassle then ensued between Mr. Lawson and my accountant, wherein he attempted to prove to Lawson that because I did not occupy a private office in a medical arts building and did not have to pay a secretary I was entitled to at least 50 percent of my house expense to compensate for this. Unfortunately, my accountant lost this battle which meant I would have to pay back taxes, plus a penalty from the time I moved into the house I built.

Lawson then began another line of questioning. He said, "Dr. Shane, do you ever visit your in-laws on Sunday?" I answered affirmatively.

"Do you travel by automobile or do you walk?"

"By automobile, of course." I answered.

"Then you do use your automobile for personal use, aside from your professional use of it, do you not?"

"Of course I do," I answered, again wondering to what he was referring.

"Dr. Shane, for years now you have been deducting expenses for your car at the rate of 100 percent. The Bureau of Internal Revenue seldom permits anyone to deduct 100 percent of an automobile, and you even admit that you use it for non-professional purposes."

Once again I directed Mr. Lawson to my accountant, explaining again that the schedule of deductions I left entirely to him, and he should certainly know what he's doing. I saw the crimson glow of embarrassment rise from the accountant's neck, and slowly engulf his countenance, his ears becoming especially red. The accountant countered in a rage, and with both barrels blazing, attempted to overwhelm the investigator with facts, figures and legal decisions, and as prejudiced as I was in my own favor, I could see almost immediately how wrong my accountant was and I began to wonder just what a financial fiasco he had gotten me into. Could this accountant be that stupid? Could an LLB and CPA be so totally uncognizant of simple, elementary law and arithmetic? Finally, after much haggling, the investigator told me directly that I would be lucky if Internal Revenue would permit me to deduct 25 percent of my automobile and that in the meantime I would have to pay at least 75 percent of delinquent taxes on automobile expenses, plus a penalty.

After winning these two points which I saw was going to cost me a considerable sum of money, Mr. Lawson began questioning me about every aspect of my work, travel, writing and even questioned the number of children I was claiming as a deduction; having been so triumphant in his previous line of questioning.

He asked me if I kept an expense account relative to the travelling I had done. I answered this in the negative, and he said, "How will you ever prove that you ever travelled?" This really had me worried.

The interview was finally over but Mr. Lawson indicated that he wanted to see all my books and cancelled checks for five years past plus a list of all sources of income and how much from each source for all those years and every item of expense; including all expenses I incurred during the building of my house.

By the time we left the Federal Building I had lost complete faith in the accountant who kept telling me not to worry about anything, it was just routine. But this routine was appearing more expensive by the minute.

Several weeks later, I received another call from Internal Revenue, this time from a man who introduced himself as special-agent Harris who wanted to question me in person at the hospital. The meeting was arranged for the next day.

In the meantime I called my accountant to apprise him of Harris' call. My accountant, whom I shall call Ellsworth, sounded somewhat apprehensive when he told me that a special agent assigned to a tax case meant that the situation had become somewhat serious and that the case was no longer a simple routine check, but was being investigated from the standpoint of possible fraud.

He told me not to worry about anything, it would all work peacefully in the end. I doubted Ellsworth's reassurance, much as I needed to believe in him, since my confidence in his tax judgment had been so severely undermined by the investigator.

A peculiar feeling began to clutch at my abdomen. It came on slowly at first, hardly noticeable. Then it began to increase in intensity. I was to become entangled in my own web of anxiety from which I could find no escape for almost two years. When special agent Harris arrived at the Lutheran Hospital the next afternoon I was in a state of near physical exhaustion from apprehension. I knew I personally had done nothing wrong. Yet I was as responsible for my tax returns as my accountant, and perhaps more so. A more severe penalty had recently been added to the

Federal Code wherein the term of imprisonment was made five years instead of one year if the government could prove fraud or intent in a tax case. The newspapers were full of stories of individuals being sent to prison or of being indicted and severely fined in Federal Court for income tax evasion, either of which would have been a public disgrace to me and my family. How many other errors did Ellsworth make on my tax returns through the years which could easily be construed as fraud? And the surgeons with whom I discussed the problem did not help matters at all. They told me that the government will frequently indict some unfortunate individual, especially when it does not involve too large a sum of money, simply as a public example for purposes of deterrence.

A Baltimore surgeon had recently been made just such an example. The more I looked at my own case the more convinced I became that I was going to be that second example. And when special agent Harris finally ended the interview I knew I was going to be the one.

I escorted Harris and another agent who accompanied him to an empty room in the surgical suite. We sat on chairs and leaned on the neat, clean bed spread. When I first saw Harris and shook hands with him I was somewhat relieved since I recognized him as a student who attended City College with me back in the thirties, although he was in none of my classes. He immediately recognized me and recalled that he had seen me in one of City's plays. The good fortune of having such a friendly special agent investigate me was such a relief that I fairly beamed with happiness. But I had appraised the warmth of our introduction a bit hastily. This man, whom I persisted in visualizing as a dishevelled, awkward youth at City College soon revealed himself to be a surly, vituperative tiger whose sole goal in life was to obtain an indictment. He wanted only to prove what he was assigned to prove: that I had committed fraud, and that ultimately I had to be sent to prison. Before five minutes had elapsed I knew that this inhuman animal was after a pound of my flesh and that nothing would deter him. The change in his character was chameleon-like as he opened his briefcase and launched into the questioning.

First he "swore me in" and reminded me that whatever I said could be used against me in Federal Court. He explained that my case had been assigned to the fraud investigation unit of The Bureau of Internal Revenue and that's why he was here.

For the record he asked me to state my name and address in the presence of his lieutenant who was his witness. He then began to question me about every aspect of my life since entering the practice of anesthesia, jotting down my answers to many of the questions. The grueling grilling lasted almost two hours and when he was finished he directed me to obtain affidavits from all the doctors I visited during my travels, receipts of all expenditures incident to the construction of my house, the names of all banks, with which I had ever dealt, the names of all hospitals and dentists or physician's offices in which I had ever administered anesthesia, and a host of other impossible-to-obtain receipts and affidavits. He warned me that he would call on me at any time and before departing told me that he would have this interview transcribed, and would send me a copy for my signature.

As revolted as I was by his demeanor (did the U.S. Government have to employ such obnoxious representatives?) I felt I had to cooperate with him for to behave otherwise might indicate guilt on my part.

After Harris and his associate departed I experienced a sensation of weight on my chest, dryness of the mouth, tachycardia and utter and devastating depression. The sight of a bird on the wing lighting on a tree just outside the hospital window made me envy the winged creature who never had to experience entangling webs of human wretchedness and anxiety. For the second time in my life I knew what fear meant. This was not fear of the dark, or fear of failing an examination or fear of losing a job. This was the kind of fear a man experiences when he awaits the gallows, having been condemned to death. I could not dispel this feeling of utter doom. I often used to think of how ridiculous it was for an individual to live a life of self-inflicted disgrace because of some infraction of the law in a specific community when all he had to do was leave the community and start anew. Such an escape from reality is so simple and uncomplicated in the realm of imagination and fantasy. But in actual day-to-day life, when a man has four children whom he loves, and lives in a house he built with his own hands, to escape by fleeing from this to a voluntary exile in some remote, even exotic land, is worse punishment than facing the investigation, the evolution of which could also result in complete innocence, rather than prison. For reasons such as this a man faces the investigation and prays for release.

I did not accompany my enemies to the hospital entrance. I saw no reason for extending any courtesy to them whatsoever. Instead, I sat and gazed out the window, in an attempt to define the uncontrollable pain which seemed to be grinding relentlessly just beneath the xiphoid process. The sensations and reactions which envelope us under differing emotional situations are themselves fascinating. In the midst of my miserable anxiety, I thought momentarily of this new pain in my upper abdomen which I had heretofore never experienced. I viewed myself as a dispassionate onlooker attempting to analyse and define this uncontrollable sensation. It was totally different from that which I experienced in dental school when all the other students received an envelope with an announcement card of graduation and I received the same envelope and the same size announcement card but mine informed me that I had failed J. Ben Robinson's course in dental history and as a consequence I was not be graduated. This note produced a devastating shock reaction but there was something I could do about it, and I did. But this income tax investigation paralyzed me. There was nothing I could do but wait. Wait and hope. But could I endure the pain and anxiety and helplessness of waiting?

Never had I experienced such a feeling of devastating doom. And as the minutes ticked by it grew worse and worse. Soon my head began to throb, then an ache commenced in my forehead and began to hammer at my temples. And all of this was totally beyond my control. I could neither dispel nor exorcise it. I felt that I could not unburden this agony on Suzi and torture her also. I left the room to phone Ellsworth. He was not in. It required codeine, aspirin and phenobarbital to give my soul a semblance of peace. I found myself projecting in empathy with small children playing on the city streets as I drove home from the hospital, envying their free minds and lack of mental anxiety. Food I could not eat, yet hunger-type pains racked me inwardly. I found subsequent relief by dosing myself with antacid emollients and realized how simple it would be to develop a stomach ulcer if I permitted this situation to continue.

The next day at noon I phoned Ellsworth who informed me that special agent Harris had spent the morning with him, and that things looked bad. I asked how bad and when Ellsworth, who was himself a lawyer, told me he had to get his own lawyer to advise him, I realized I would have to get my own lawyer to advise me and that Ellsworth was apparently in trouble himself which did my cause and my internal environment no good whatsoever! Ellsworth's depression immediately reflected itself on my already anxiety-ridden mind. it was almost too much to bear. The only one on whom I could unburden myself was Buzzy, my brother, who advised me to obtain the best tax lawyer in Baltimore, regardless of the cost. I had been burned by one so-called tax lawyer and my faith in individuals of this ilk left me cold.

The investigation meanwhile continued. Doctors began to corner me in the corridors or out in the hospital parking lot, and in very discreet whispers each warned me, as if he were the only one, that he had received a visit by an agent of The U.S. Treasury Department, making inquiries about me, wanting to know if and when I ever administered anesthesia for any of these men in institutions outside the Lutheran Hospital. It became so widespread that as soon as a doctor indicated he wanted to speak with me in private, away from all third persons, I knew that another cop of the Internal Revenue special-agent division had flashed his badge in another doctor's office.

Unless one personally experiences this severe degree of harassment by an organization as all-powerful as the U.S. Government it is impossible to realize the degree of physical pain which continuous and unrelenting anxiety, fear and apprehension may cause.

The fact of this ruthless, unnecessary investigation hounded me literally to death for almost two years. There were incessant calls from the supersnooper Harris, asking for this receipt; did I recall that item of expense, did I ever visit Dr. So and So? There were calls from surgeons and dentists wanting to know what in the world was going on.

I finally did what my brother suggested. I went to a lawyer named Edward Houck, who himself for twenty years was chief of the special agents division of Internal Revenue. In fact, Houck had at one time been Harris' boss prior to his leaving the Bureau and going into private law practice.

When I explained the situation to Houck he said to me, "You know, Dr. Shane, I've spent the past twenty years trying to put income tax evaders into prison, and now I spend my time trying to keep them out. And keeping them out is far more lucrative than sending them up."

I liked Houck and I liked the way he worked. The first thing he did after legally obtaining all my records from my accountant was to determine whether or not there was fraud in any aspect of my tax returns. When he was convinced there was none he ordered special agent Harris up to his office to see him. Houck told me that when Harris came to his office he was like a docile child who stood in awe before a domineering parent. After I explained the situation to Houck, and showed him that my entire awkward position was due entirely to an ignorant, misguided, so-called tax attorney, Houck then interviewed Ellsworth, became convinced that I was not at fault in any respect, and within one month settled the entire case without any fraudulent association being placed on my record.

Ellsworth, meanwhile, was fired from his accountancy organization and lost his privilege to practice before the tax courts. He died within a year.

When Houck finally called me and announced that the investigation was over and that the case had been settled the weight of the universe was suddenly lifted from my shoulders. I don't recall when I ever felt so happy, so lighthearted, so full of song. For the first time in two years the leaves appeared green again; I saw once more the blue of the sky. The sound of birds in the morning was again a symphony, and I became one with birds and children and other free and kindred spirits. How beautiful life suddenly became. How sweet was the world. Although they did not know it, I had incarcerated myself for two years because of an immature cop named Harris who derived a morbid sense of satisfaction and power from flashing his Treasury Department badge.

During this two-year nightmare of silent, introspective agony, I developed a sensation of constriction in my throat which grew in intensity each time I was paged for a phone call at the hospital. The sensation varied from day to day but it was always there. Hot tea or coffee seemed to relieve it temporarily and so did an ounce of Jack Daniels. But I shall never forget the day that Houck phoned me and informed me that the case was settled. My throat from that second on seemed to be released from an iron constricting band which no amount of rationalization, attempted self-hypnosis, long soliloquies with myself could ever obliterate. I could swallow again without discomfort. I had had two throat specialists examine me because of this. Once again I was able to see demonstrated on myself as a guinea pig, that anxiety and aggravation can result in psychosomatic manifestations which are real, and which actually exist and which are definitely not imaginary.

I was left with a peculiar residual after this experience. I observed that on an occasion when I found myself under severe strain or tension the same band of constricting tightness returned to my throat, making swallowing difficult and actually producing considerable discomfort. Having further observed the disease was cured instantly with the mentally allieviating phone call from Houck, I would then apply this psychological remedy to the tension of the moment; stare it in the face; dissect its cause with brutal honesty; and having overcome the tension my throat, would return to normal. The cure which I could produce in myself by this method of honest self-analysis and introspection was almost miraculous. And I am certain that ulcers of the digestive tract and other physical manifestation of anxiety can be similarly obviated.

EPILOGUE

As this book goes to press I am about to enter my 70th year. I have been to almost every nook and cranny of this earth and have sailed the seven seas. I have sensed the heat of the Equator in Africa and the unbelievable cold of Antarctica. No continent is a stranger to my presence.

At 70 I have left remaining, at the most, 30 more years of individual days. Since I have already experienced the disappearance of two thirty-year epochs plus ten, I know how swiftly they can dissolve into the evanescent film of memories.

Since some of my life's experiences were unusual I decided to record them in this book. My experiences in the Northwest Passage, the anesthesia years at Johns Hopkins, the details of building a house with my own hands, exploring the Baja of Mexico, and the detailed experience of a major operation in the 20th Century may have some historical value in the decades ahead.

My eleven grandchildren and their progeny will ultimately be the most appreciative of this effort. I therefore humbly dedicate and leave this legacy of requited dreams to those of my great grandchildren yet unborn.

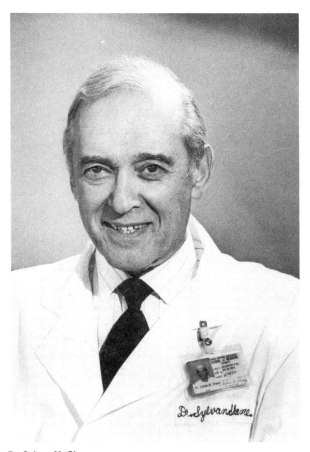

Dr. Sylvan M. Shane.

ABOUT THE AUTHOR

WAR AGAINST TIME is the author's 12th book. Dr. Shane, an anesthesiologist and a dentist, was born in Baltimore in 1918, was educated at the University of Southern California and was graduated from the Johns Hopkins University and the University of Maryland School of Dentistry in 1943. He was an Assistant Professor of Anesthesiology and Critical Care Medicine at the Johns Hopkins University School of Medicine until his retirement in 1984, then returned to teach on a part time basis. He was the recipient of the Heidbrink Anesthesia Award for his research contributions to ambulatory anesthetics. He has circled the world three times lecturing on his specialty, and this book is a compendium of his observations in the form of 11 essays. Dr. Shane is the father of four children who have produced eleven grandchildren. He resides in Westminister, Maryland on a six acre hill, in a glass house, which he built with his own hands.